Krav Maga for Beginners

Krav Maga for Beginners

A Step-by-Step Guide to the World's Easiest-to-Learn, Most-Effective Fitness and Fighting Program

DARREN LEVINE
JOHN WHITMAN
RYAN HOOVER

Photographs by Andy Mogg

Ulysses Press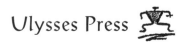

In memory of Marni

———————

Published in the United States by
ULYSSES PRESS
P.O. Box 3440
Berkeley, CA 94703
www.ulyssespress.com

ISBN: 978-1-56975-661-4
Library of Congress Control Number 2007907807

Printed in Canada by Webcom

10 9 8 7 6 5 4 3 2 1

Contributing writer	Kevin Lewis
Acquisitions	Nick Denton-Brown
Editorial/Production	Lily Chou, Claire Chun, Lauren Harrison, Katy Loveless
Index	Sayre Van Young
Design	what!design @ whatweb.com
Cover photographs	Andy Mogg
Interior photographs	Andy Mogg except on page 8 © Krav Maga Worldwide, Inc.
Models	Tina Angelotti, Kelly Ann Campbell, Shannon Castro, Jeanine Jackson, Kirian Fitzgibbons, Ryan Hoover, Gabriel Khorramian, Marcus Kowal, Darren Levine, Kevin Lewis, Kokushi Matsumoto, Karla Nystrom, Matthew Romond, Jessen San Luis, John Whitman

Visit Krav Maga Worldwide online at www.kravmaga.com

Distributed by Publishers Group West

Please Note
This book has been written and published strictly for informational purposes, and in no way should be used as a substitute for actual instruction with qualified professionals. The author and publisher are providing you with information in this work so that you can have the knowledge and can choose, at your own risk, to act on that knowledge. The author and publisher also urge all readers to be aware of their health status and to consult health care professionals before beginning any health program.

Table of Contents

DEFENSES

GROUNDFIGHTING

Purpose of This Book

Krav Maga for Beginners is meant to be a prequel to *Complete Krav Maga*. We published that book with the intent of providing a complete, detailed, and useful guide to the Krav Maga curriculum as presented by Krav Maga Worldwide. It covers every technique from yellow belt through brown belt—essentially, the first five levels of the system.

But we realized, after the fact, that we'd given some beginners a book that was too broad and not deep enough. We decided to go back and write a book that focuses on the first two levels of the system (yellow and orange). This book provides not only the physical description of techniques, but additional teaching points and commonly asked questions. So while *Complete Krav Maga* is a detailed manual you can follow, *Krav Maga for Beginners* is almost like having an instructor there to answer some of your questions, or to tell you why we do things the way we do.

That last part is important to us. We never want Krav Maga techniques to be done simply because we told you to. There should be a reason behind every specific movement and, if there isn't a reason, then that movement should be open to whatever interpretation you want to make.

We challenge our students to ask us "why?" in every class because that's how we all grow. Often, we can provide answers that satisfy those questions in logical ways. But every now and then, a student asks a question that makes us think—a question that opens a new door and maybe even improves and simplifies a technique.

Who knows? Maybe you'll be that student.

What Is Krav Maga?

Krav Maga is not pretty. It's not elegant either, and it certainly isn't an "art" in the way most people think of traditional martial arts. While there is absolutely nothing wrong with training in more graceful systems such as wing chun kung fu or tai chi, the Krav Maga defensive tactics systems leave all that beauty at the doorstep and goes out into the street to train in simple, aggressive movements that get right to the point of self-defense.

Krav Maga (pronounced *kräv mägä*), which is Hebrew for "close combat," was originally developed by Imi Lichtenfeld for the Israeli military, which needed a hand-to-hand combat system that could be learned quickly and would be effective regardless of age, gender, athletic attributes, or body type. Krav Maga was developed in a hostile environment in which combatants could not devote many hours to hand-to-hand combat training. There are no forms or rules or set combinations as reactions to attacks. Krav Maga training focuses on teaching simple self-defense techniques based on the body's natural reactions.

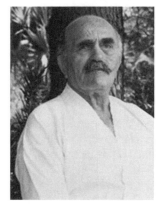

Krav Maga, as opposed to many other systems or styles, is a survival system dealing with personal safety issues. It is a modern, highly refined self-defense method designed to be used against both unarmed and armed attackers, as well as multiple assailants.

Krav Maga is based on principles rather than specific techniques. This is an important distinction, because systems which are technique-driven do not allow for the possibility of variations in attacks, reactions to counterattacks, body types, physical limitations, environment, and other variables that will likely be present in a violent encounter.

Imi Lichtenfeld, the founder of Krav Maga.

Krav Maga is an integrated system, which means techniques that are taught will be applicable in more than one situation, allowing students to learn a few responses to many different attacks. Krav Maga is not simply an amalgamation of other arts and styles, but a carefully assembled and researched system that allows for congruence throughout, from very basic to very advanced levels.

Krav Maga is battle-tested, and Krav Maga involves pressure-testing students in training in order to improve survivability "in the streets." Stress drills are vital to the training and pressure-testing process. The drills are designed to replicate, as closely as possible, the stress of violent conflict through mental, physical, and emotional challenges.

Krav Maga Worldwide's popularity in the global community continues to grow as more and more people find it to be the ideal combination of practical, real-world self-defense and a challenging and fun fitness alternative. Over 200 law enforcement agencies have adopted Krav Maga training, and with over 200 affiliated schools in the United States and continued growth internationally, Krav Maga Worldwide is the preeminent source for Krav Maga training.

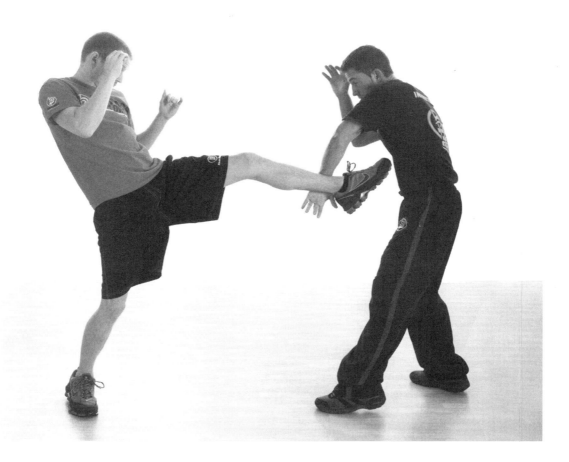

Is Krav Maga Right for Me?

The principal objective of Krav Maga is to get practitioners, regardless of age, size, or gender, to a level of self-defense proficiency in a relatively short period of time. While designed for soldiers with little time for hand-to-hand combat training, the methods and techniques used in Krav Maga are a perfect fit for the busy lifestyles of today's citizens, who do not have the time or inclination to devote years to training.

Krav Maga works for everyone. An effective self-defense system cannot rely solely on physical attributes. Krav Maga was designed for a military that enlists citizens of all ages, sizes, and genders, so explosive movements were incorporated into the system. These movements mitigate an attacker's ability to adjust to the defense. Krav Maga also employs the use of strikes to vulnerable areas of an attacker, like eyes, throat, and groin, which can produce maximum damage with minimum effort.

Krav Maga does not require years of training to achieve self-defense proficiency. Krav Maga training today has been further refined to meet the needs of citizens and law enforcement personnel with other endeavors and responsibilities in daily life. Krav Maga is perfect for adults with limited training time and a desire for an enhanced quality of life and an increased sense of security and self-confidence. Krav Maga's training methodology allows students to achieve all of these goals in a relatively short period of time.

Krav Maga is strictly self-defense and fitness for adults. Many adults today are not interested in the formalities of traditional martial arts. The purposes of Krav Maga are simply self-defense and fitness, so training time is spent cultivating those goals. Typical classes consist of warm-ups, combatives training, self-defense techniques, and stress drills. Training time is devoted only to enhancing survivability in a violent encounter. In Krav Maga, it is important that your training matches your goals, and the training is performed in an environment conducive to achieving those goals.

Krav Maga is a great way to get into shape and relieve stress. Many actors, such as Jennifer Lopez, Brendan Fraser, Kristanna Loken, Lucy Liu, Jennifer Garner, Leonardo Di Caprio, Dennis Haysbert, Brad Pitt, and Hilary Swank, have sought out Krav Maga training as a way to enhance their on-screen fighting prowess and physique. As more and more people are looking for a unique and exciting way to get into shape while getting out of the gym and off of the treadmill, many are finding that Krav Maga classes fit the bill. The classes are also a fantastic way to relieve the stress that often accompanies a hectic lifestyle. Krav Maga training utilizes functional exercise regimens to tone, shape, strengthen, and further condition the body and mind. This prepares students for violent encounters on the street, stressful mornings in the boardroom, or even extra-demanding days with the kids.

Where You Can Train in Krav Maga

Krav Maga Worldwide, at the printing of this book, recognizes over 240 officially licensed training facilities worldwide. These training centers are required to have certified instructors teaching the Krav Maga classes, and the centers and instructors are held to very high training and teaching standards. The certification process is very demanding, with 30 to 40 percent of instructor candidates failing the initial phase of training.

For an updated listing of these centers, please visit the locations page of the Krav Maga Worldwide website at www.kravmaga.com.

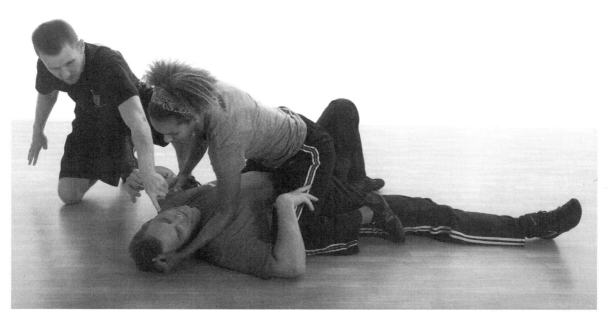

Author Ryan Hoover points out a vulnerable point on the attacker.

Krav Maga Philosophy and
Principles

Krav Maga is ultimately about problem solving, and while its original purpose was to address violent encounters, the same philosophy can be applied to other facets of daily life. Krav Maga is a no-nonsense, no-frills system that is designed to instill a fighting spirit and aggressive mindset in its students. While Krav Maga recognizes that self-defense is not punishment, and that the ultimate goal is to go home safely, the tenets dictate that the best way to achieve that goal is to react aggressively and decisively.

Don't get hurt. While this may seem obvious, the intent is far-reaching. This tenet dictates that great lengths should be taken to avoid conflict if at all possible. Often, an improved understanding of the dynamics of violence and violent people will heighten awareness and avoidance. However, if this is not possible, it is imperative that the defender is aggressive in order to eliminate the threat and neutralize the attacker, diminishing the chances for injury.

Train from a position of disadvantage. Life, by its very nature, makes even the most vigilant trainee prone to distraction. Whether it is a mental lapse, complacency, or worse, apathy, lapses are natural. Krav Maga training takes such realities into consideration and forces students to train from a poor state of readiness. Understanding that it is highly probable that a defender will be forced to take action when unprepared, training is typically conducted from a neutral position. This position forces the student to perform techniques without regard to proper footwork, hand positioning, balance, weight distribution, etc. In order for Krav Maga to be the most effective for reality, the techniques and tactics must not rely on being early in the defense or prepared. This is a significant element of Krav Maga training.

Identify and eliminate the immediate danger. Without addressing the true problem, no "technique" or "resolution" can be successful. Often, valuable time is lost while peripheral issues are addressed. Krav Maga

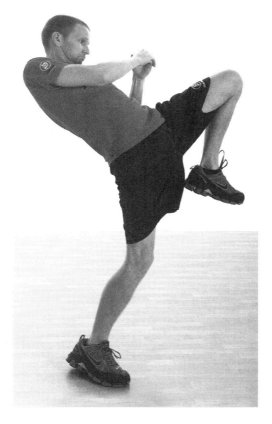

stresses that the most imminent danger must be taken care of first, and that it should be done in the most efficient fashion.

Utilize the body's natural instincts. While other styles or systems may teach techniques that some may deem "better" under given circumstances, most often these techniques work against the body's natural reactions and require extensive time in training. Techniques such as these are entirely less likely to work under the stress of a violent encounter.

Krav Maga recognizes that fine motor skills are much less effective under the influence of the adrenaline that accompanies stressful situations, so techniques are gross motor by design and draw heavily from what the body would most likely do naturally. This approach increases the likelihood of performing a technique successfully during the stress of a real-life violent encounter. It also lessens the amount of training time needed to achieve a reasonable level of proficiency.

For the average person, and that is the focus, copious training is not practical. Krav Maga training takes into account that the body's response to violence or fear falls into three categories, typically described as fight, flight, or freeze. This training incorporates drills that encourage decisive reaction under stress, taking the defender from a state of inaction to a state of action quickly.

Deal effectively with secondary dangers that may exist in the attack. Understanding that identifying and eliminating the immediate threat in any attack is paramount to a successful defense, it is also necessary to consider secondary dangers that may result as an extension of the attack or as a by-product of the defense. Secondary dangers are most effectively mitigated through the use of sound tactics and application of the other key principles, such as being explosive and defending and countering simultaneously.

Counterattack as soon as possible, preferably simultaneously to the defense. A strong counterattack is vital to any realistic defense. A strong and aggressive counter is designed to disrupt the ongoing attack. It forces the attacker to react to the defender, as opposed to continuing or adjusting the attack. The sooner this attack is delivered, the quicker the defender is able to shift the "predator vs. prey" paradigm. Remember, virtually all criminals are looking for a victim, not a fight, so an aggressive and immediate counter will also serve to surprise the attacker, creating openings for further counters and escape. Defense does not "win" an altercation!

Attack vulnerable areas. Again, a viable self-defense system must not be based on the defender's physical attributes. Therefore, Krav Maga emphasizes attacking to vulnerable areas, such as the eyes, jaw, throat, liver, kidneys, groin, fingers, knees, shins, and insteps. Strikes to these areas allow defenders to do maximum damage with minimal effort and strength.

Analyze and use the environment whenever possible. Violent attacks rarely occur in a controlled environment. Krav Maga emphasizes the need to evaluate the environment in order to choose the proper action. As an example, if defending on uneven, unstable, or slippery terrain, upper body strikes are often preferred over kicks.

Training also encourages the use of common objects found on the scene, either offensively (e.g., blunt object for striking) or defensively (e.g., chair as a shield), in order to increase the chances of surviving an attack. This is extremely important since fights are rarely "fair." If someone is intent on doing harm, the defender must do whatever is necessary, using whatever is available (lamp, bottle, plate, briefcase, fire extinguisher, electrical cord, etc.). This principle applies regardless of what the advantages or disadvantages appear to be in the moment. Fights are dynamic, and variables can change in an instant (introduction of weapons, third parties, injuries, etc.). Krav Maga stresses that defenders do *whatever* it takes to go home safely.

Mindset: Don't quit. A proper Krav Maga training regimen will go to great lengths, through specially designed drills, to develop a fighting spirit in each practitioner. In real situations, early recognition of potential violence and consequent variable mitigation are imperative. In times of potential danger, many factors can affect the outcome of the altercation, and most are controlled, at least initially, by the attacker. That said, the fighting spirit developed through Krav Maga training may very well be the one factor under the defender's control. Therefore, it must be nurtured and cultivated to become pervasive.

This intangible is similar to that developed in many militaries—a term known as cognitive dissonance, or, in short, the concept that attitude follows behavior. Krav Maga drills physically empower and consequently emotionally empower its students. The systematic process of training under new and varied stressors serves to galvanize the skill set needed to perform in times of actual duress.

The essence of Krav Maga, and what will save the defender, is the willingness to do whatever it takes to survive. The philosophy that a "never say die" attitude can be strengthened through training is the linchpin that allows Krav Maga students to adapt under the most stressful situation and emerge successfully from violent confrontations, regardless of the dynamic.

Flee to safety. Ultimately, the goal is to go home safely. Krav Maga training stresses that it is critically important to defend aggressively to insure that the threat is no longer viable. That said, it is simultaneously important to avoid remaining in harm's way longer than is required. As time elapses, variables (introduction of weapons, additional attackers, fatigue, injury, etc.) increase, therefore the defender should look to leave the scene as soon as safely possible. Remember, violent encounters are unique, and the situation will dictate the response, including the time to safely escape.

Never do more than is necessary. As previously stated, the goal of Krav Maga training is to enhance survivability. Krav Maga, out of necessity, is an aggressive and forceful system. However, these are adjectives used to describe a self-defense system, and self-defense should never become punishment.

Eliminating the threat means doing just enough to facilitate escape. As a defender, it is not acceptable to exact punishment or vengeance on the attacker. This is not only morally unacceptable; more importantly, it is tactically unsound, since the defender runs the risk of staying engaged longer than necessary, increasing the chances of other variables coming into play. Often, extrication is the best solution.

Krav Maga and Fitness

Fitness, as it relates to Krav Maga, must be combat functional. In other words, the exercises, drills, and methods used are designed to enhance physical tools important for improving self-defense performance. Exercises closely replicate movements involved in self-defense training, and the exercises are goal specific. Combat functional fitness, for the purpose of Krav Maga training, must address, at a minimum, strength training, explosiveness, stamina, and flexibility.

The unique training methods of Krav Maga have often allowed students to achieve physiques, confidence, and fitness levels never before realized. As self-defense professionals, the goal of Krav Maga instructors is to make students safer. As opposed to typical gym fitness programs, Krav Maga offers life-saving techniques and tactics to go with the newly sculpted bodies.

Strength Training
The goal of strength training, unlike bodybuilding, is not aesthetics. Strength training is solely about increasing strength, not about increasing size or cultivating a look. Strength training focuses on developing or enhancing athletic attributes, and while there are many means with which to improve strength, for the purposes of Krav Maga training, some are preferred over others.

Strength, as it relates to Krav Maga goals, serves to augment a student's capacity to cause damage to an attacker as well as absorb punishment. While Krav Maga strongly emphasizes the need for aggressive counter-attacks, Krav Maga instruction also focuses on performing from a position of disadvantage, which may involve defending after being struck or while being struck.

Explosiveness
Explosiveness is the ability to produce maximum effort or strength in a short amount of time. While closely related to strength training, being strong does not equal explosive. Exercises to develop explosiveness are com-

monly referred to as plyometrics, where the goal is to increase the amount of force applied and decrease the time needed to apply it.

In most Krav Maga defenses, the ability to perform explosively is the great equalizer. Because the force is dispatched rapidly, as opposed to gradually, explosive reactions aid to mitigate an attacker's ability to adjust to defenses and counters. This is an important aspect of Krav Maga, since it allows smaller defenders to perform against larger defenders.

Flexibility

Krav Maga does not rely on or emphasize fancy techniques, but flexibility, when defined as increased range of motion, is important for reaching maximum potential in all techniques, particularly combatives. Range of motion is typically described as the distance that can be achieved between the flexed position and the extended position of specific muscle groups or joints. Increasing flexibility helps to reduce injuries, as well as increase power and speed, by allowing joints and muscles to fully extend.

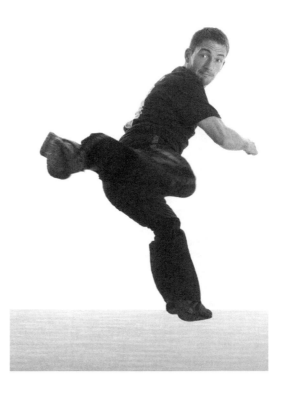

Endurance

Endurance or stamina is the ability to exert maximum or near-maximum effort through aerobic or anaerobic training over an extended period of time. While most violent encounters last less than a minute, endurance training is an essential aspect of a complete functional fitness program. The stress that accompanies a violent encounter, coupled with the necessary physical response to the attack, will cause the body to rapidly fatigue. Recognizing this, fitness training must include a focus on endurance and must condition the body and mind to exert maximum effort for as long as is necessary to eliminate the threat and facilitate escape. Furthermore, since violent situations are tense, uncertain, and rapidly evolving, the dynamics of the encounter may change, and the introduction of new threats will require the stamina to continue fighting.

The History of Krav Maga in the United States

While many people in the United States were first exposed to Krav Maga in the Jennifer Lopez movie *Enough*, it has been in the United States since 1981. This was the year the Krav Maga Association of Israel, headed by Imi Lichtenfeld, and the Israeli Ministry of Education held the first International Instructors Course for Krav Maga through the Wingate Institute for Physical Education and Sport.

A philanthropist from New York, S. Daniel Abraham, sponsored a delegation of 23 members from various cities in the United States to attend the course, which was supervised by Imi himself. Imi was 71 years old at the time and retired from his military career. Darren Levine was selected to be a part of the delegation because of his martial arts and boxing background, as well as his involvement in the physical education program at the Heschel Day School in the San Fernando Valley, California.

The instructor's course was an intensive six-week course consisting of eight hours of training during the day and additional hours of optional training at night. The students trained six days a week. During the six weeks, Imi befriended Darren. At the conclusion of the course, Imi told Darren that he would spend the following summer in Los Angeles teaching and training him. It was a strenuous and exhausting six weeks and, by the end of the course, only six members, including Darren, passed.

Darren began teaching Krav Maga at the Heschel Day School as an elective class, but by 1982, the class had become so popular that it was incorporated into the physical education program. The popularity also brought about a separate, evening adult program, focusing on self-defense, fighting, and cutting-edge fitness. In the summer of 1982, true to his word, Imi came to Los Angeles and spent many weeks with Darren and his family while instructing Darren in Krav Maga, as well as teaching children and adults alongside Darren.

In 1983, at Imi's urging, Darren, with the help of prominent members of the Jewish community, including Joel Bernstein and Mark Lainer, formed the Krav Maga Association of America, Inc. The goals of this organization were to regulate and promote Krav Maga in the United States, as well as to help promote good relations between the United States and Israel.

Every summer after Imi's visit, Darren would either go to Israel to train in Krav Maga, or Imi himself would return or send a top military or civilian instructor to the United States to train Darren. At the end of 1984, Darren received his first-degree black belt in Krav Maga. At Darren's belt award ceremony, Imi's black belt was passed on to him. Darren also received his full instructor teaching certification from the Wingate Institute for Physical Education and Sport and the Krav Maga Association of Israel that same year. In 1985, Imi penned a letter recognizing Darren as an expert in Krav Maga.

Through the Krav Maga Association of America, Darren and his top students began teaching Krav Maga to law enforcement in the United States. Darren also worked to adapt Krav Maga to suit the needs of U.S. peace and military officers. Imi came back to the United States in 1987 to help Darren teach Krav Maga to the Illinois State Police, and in 1988, Imi and Colonel David Ben-Asher co-wrote yet another letter identifying Darren as an expert in Krav Maga for law enforcement.

Darren continued to teach Krav Maga at Heschel until 1987, when he moved the classes to the University of Judaism. Classes at the University of Judaism continued until 1996, when demand for Krav Maga was so great that the Krav Maga National Training Center was opened in West Los Angeles. It was the first center of its kind, blending Krav Maga with a fitness program and establishing a training ground for civilians and law enforcement personnel that previously had never existed anywhere in the world.

Imi was quite proud of the growth and success of Krav Maga in the U.S. In 1997, shortly after Darren received his sixth-degree black belt in Krav Maga, Imi awarded Darren a Founder's Diploma for Special Excellence in Krav Maga. Imi gave this diploma to only two individuals, Darren and Eyal Yanilov, the Director of the International Krav Maga Federation. These diplomas were given to the people that Imi wanted to be the leaders of Krav Maga.

In January 1999, Krav Maga Worldwide Enterprises was formed to facilitate the expansion of the Krav Maga system throughout the U.S. and around the world. Imi, through his words and actions, viewed Darren Levine as the person most capable and qualified to develop techniques, train instructors, and adapt Krav Maga based on the needs of American citizens and law enforcement agencies. As a result, Krav Maga Worldwide, under the expert direction of Mr. Levine, has successfully maintained the integrity of the Krav Maga system and principles, as intended by Imi. Krav Maga Worldwide has also been responsible for keeping Krav Maga relevant and up to date, specifically for the unique and changing needs of the citizens of the United States and other industrialized nations.

Krav Maga Worldwide has had great success in exposing Krav Maga to hundreds of thousands of people throughout the world, while also getting the system approved and recognized for use by more than 200 law enforcement agencies. Krav Maga Worldwide is also intimately involved in training some of the U.S. military's most elite units. Krav Maga continues to thrive in the U.S. and abroad, and it is the objective of Krav Maga Worldwide to continue to present the best in self-defense training to as many people as possible.

Important Considerations

Once you've made the decision to begin your Krav Maga training, there are several items to keep in mind to insure the best training experience. Hopefully, you're able to find a certified Krav Maga Worldwide instructor (see page 11 for more information), and your instructor will be sure to speak to these considerations as well.

Preparing for a Training Session

In order to get the most out of your sessions, you should be prepared, physically and mentally, for the training. You should consult your physician to insure that this type of training is suitable for you.

As part of your physical preparations, you should consider a diet that will optimize your session. Eating a carbohydrate-rich meal three to four hours before training will serve to fuel your body. Eating an easily digestible snack an hour or so beforehand should give you the added boost to get you started. Since most Krav Maga sessions last an hour, water is ideal for your hydration. It's important to drink water, not only during your training, but throughout the day.

A typical Krav Maga Worldwide class consists of a warm-up (see page 37 for details), combatives training, self-defense training, and drills. Warm-ups are designed to prepare the body both physically and mentally for the hard training ahead, but you know your body better than anyone. If you have problem areas that need extra attention (such as stretching), you should take the initiative to address this before your session begins. It's also imperative that you notify your instructor of any injuries that you may have.

You should also spend some preparation time on getting ready mentally. As is done on the physical side, your certified instructor will employ techniques to do just this, but you should spend some time thinking about the training and your training goals before you begin the class. Simply showing up to train is a big step, but coming in with specific goals in mind, and the understanding that maximum effort will produce maximum results, will provide you with the best training experience.

Wrapping Hands

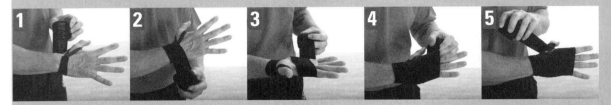

Handwraps are designed to provide wrist and knuckle protection during hard punching. While there are many ways to wrap the hands, here's a very common and practical way.

1-2 Relax your hand and spread your fingers. Place the thumb loop around your thumb and bring the wrap across the back of your hand. Wrap around your wrist two or three times, two to three inches up from your wrist joint, to insure proper support. The hand wrap should be snug, but be careful not to cut off your circulation. *Note:* The wrap should not be twisted at any point.

3 From the wrist, bring the wrap across the back of your hand and around your palm.

4 Continue the wrap across the top of your knuckles. Wrap the knuckles two to three times. Create an "X" pattern across the back of your hand by starting at the knuckles and going across the back of your hand toward your wrist and around. Replicate this "X" pattern two or three times.

Safety in Training

While your certified instructor and licensed training facility will go to great lengths to produce a safe training experience, the onus is often on the student to insure personal safety and the safety of training partners. Krav Maga Worldwide classes are designed to prepare students for self-defense in the real world. The recommended training attire reflects this goal, while also making considerations for optimal training. Lightweight nylon pants or knee-length shorts are preferred, along with a T-shirt and cross-training-type shoes. It's also essential, in order to maintain a safe training environment and as a courtesy to fellow students, to keep these items clean. Bringing extra shirts, in order to change during or between classes, is a common courtesy all students should make a habit.

Krav Maga Worldwide training centers attract people from all walks of life, with varying experiences, backgrounds, and training goals. It's important to understand and respect these factors when training. When partnering, students should try to partner with those of similar size. This may not always be possible, so considering potential size and strength differences to insure the safety of everyone is vital to a productive training atmosphere. While students are there to better themselves, peripheral goals should include bettering the others in the class. Also, while we want to engender a realistic training experience, this should not be done at the unnecessary risk of injury. If you feel a student does not wholly understand how to train safely, speak with your instructor.

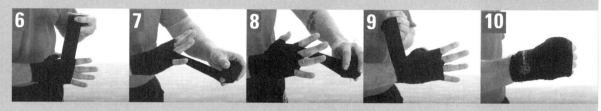

5 Continue wrapping around the palm of your hand to the bottom of your thumb. Wrap around your thumb and back toward your wrist, on the palm side. Continue to wrap around the back of your hand to the thumb. Wrap around the thumb once more (this time it will be from the opposite direction.)

6 Continue from the thumb, over the back of your hand and around your wrist.

7 Wrap around your wrist, over the back of your hand, and between your pinky and ring finger. Wrap around your palm toward your wrist. Repeat this step for all fingers, but not the thumb.

8 After the last finger, bring the wrap across the palm toward your wrist. Continue across the back of your hand, up toward your knuckles.

9 Wrap the top of the knuckles again and continue across the back of your hand toward your wrist.

10 Wrap the wrist with the remainder of the wrap, and fasten the hook and loop.

Your training environment should be controlled as much as possible. If training at a licensed facility, this should be a normal part of business, but you should do your part to be diligent in understanding inherent or potential dangers. You should remove obstacles that are not imperative to the training at hand. You should check equipment to verify its integrity. If training outdoors, be sure to scan the area and remove items that may be hazardous. If you are not training at a licensed facility, you should be sure to have a first-aid kit on hand during your sessions.

Recommended Training Equipment

Certain items are essential for the ideal training experience. For combative training, there are several types of training pads that will serve to enhance your training.

The *punch or "tombstone" pad* is very versatile. Most upper body combatives, as well as some kicks, can be performed on this pad.

The *kickshield pad* is ideal for practicing many of the stronger kicks used in Krav Maga. It's also used for practicing knees and prevalent in many training drills.

Focus mitts are used for intermediate and advanced combative training, particularly punches.

Kickshield

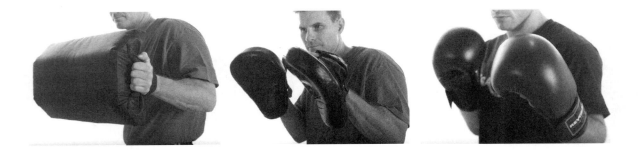

Tombstone   Focus mitts   Boxing gloves

In order to train hard and minimize injuries, there are several pieces of gear that are essential. Handwraps, gloves, mouthpieces, and groin protection are at the top of the list. However, it's also important to train, at times, without this gear. This should be done only in a controlled and supervised training environment.

There are many styles and sizes of gloves, which vary according to training goals. For basic Krav Maga training, 12- to 16-ounce boxing gloves are ideal for heavy punching and controlled sparring. These gloves may be worn with or without handwraps. While there are inexpensive options out there, the higher-quality gloves are more durable and provide more protection.

Dealing Successfully with a
Violent Encounter

Self-defense is not just about learning techniques. Violent encounters are by definition frightening, visceral events involving extreme reactions on several levels: the emotional/psychological level and the physiological level. Good training helps to prepare you for these aspects of violence.

Emotional Responses

Emotional responses to a violent encounter (or even a potentially violent encounter) include all the obvious extremes of fear (for oneself or others) and anger (at being put in danger). The wife of one of this book's authors was carjacked and recalls feeling, along with fear, a sense of outrage and confusion. She kept demanding of the carjacker, "Why are you doing this? Why?" She didn't expect a response, but her outrage demanded an answer (we'll discuss this further below in the comments on psychology). One of the authors himself was threatened with a gun (prior to learning Krav Maga) and recalls being not afraid but furious, and determined not to allow the would-be robber to succeed.

But emotional responses are usually issues to deal with after the fact, when treating oneself or others suffering from post-traumatic stress. During the violent encounter itself, emotional responses tend to be symptoms of powerful physical and psychological responses, and it is these that we will discuss in detail here.

Fight, Flight, or Freeze

The "fight or flight" response, also known as the "acute stress response," was extensively documented by Dr. Walter Cannon in the 1920s. In "fight or flight," the nervous system pumps adrenaline and norepinephrine into the body, triggering an increase in heart rate, constriction of blood vessels, and a tightening of the muscles. Essentially, the body is preparing itself for a short burst of sudden and extreme physical activity. As an interesting side note (especially for Krav Maga, which bases itself so much on instinct), an abundance of certain hormones (catecholamines) at neuroreceptor sites encourages the body to rely on spontaneous or intuitive reactions that often help during combat or evasion.*

But what, specifically, happens during the "fight or flight" response? Here are a few of the most typical physical and psychological reactions.

Physical Reactions

Essentially, during moments of intense stress, your strength goes way up and your dexterity goes way down. You experience a very short period of extreme physical ability (although you're unlikely to enjoy it!) but without much control of your fine motor skills. For this reason, any techniques you employ must avoid precise movements. In a nutshell, the following occurs:

- Increased heart rate
- Increased blood pressure
- Increased respiration
- Imperviousness to pain
- Increased strength (followed by a drastic drop)
- Increased speed
- Drastic loss of fine motor skills

Psychological Responses

Some of the most interesting (and challenging) responses to a violent, stressful encounter are psychological. Here are some of the more common:

Tachypsychia—literally, tachypsychia means "speed of the mind" and it refers to the brain's ability to perceive the passage of time under stress. In highly stressful situations, the brain kicks into high gear, absorbing information at a rapid pace. The result is that things seem to move in slow motion, even though you (and your opponent in a fight) are probably moving very fast. It's also possible for tachypsychia to happen in reverse, so that a surprised victim of assault is shocked by the speed with which events occur.

Tunnel vision—the brain becomes focused on the threat to the exclusion of all else. Peripheral vision is impaired or entirely absent and one appears to be looking down a tube or tunnel. It takes an act of will to see anything outside of this field of vision. As far as survival instincts go, tunnel vision is beneficial because it focuses the mind on the immediate threat. However, it can be a problem if you're dealing with multiple attackers or an unpredictable environment.

Auditory exclusion—or, if you prefer, "tunnel hearing." It's the aural version of tunnel vision. The mind shuts out anything that does not seem to be pertinent to immediate survival. The drawback to auditory exclusion is

---

* While "fight" and "flight" are the best-known reactions, there is a corollary of the "flight" response called "freeze." In some individuals, the physiological response is so overpowering that they simply do nothing. They shut down, simply wanting the incident to be over. This is the typical "deer in headlights" response.

We believe that whatever training you do must allow you to avoid the "freeze" response. Possums freeze. Rabbits, in certain situations, freeze, because by freezing they hope to avoid detection. But we're not talking about avoiding detection. We assume that the violent encounter has already begun. Running away (when practical) is fine. Fighting is often required. But from our point of view, freezing is not an option.

that you may not hear allies yelling at you to watch your back, or to run.

Cognitive dissonance—a fancy phrase for confusion. The brain remembers events out of sequence, and small details (the color of shoe laces, the part in someone's hair) take on great importance while major details (the type of handgun used, the color of eyes, the license plate of a car) recede and disappear.

Denial—the brain simply refuses to acknowledge the danger (this is akin to the "freeze" response mentioned in a previous footnote) or shuts down in the face of imminent injury.

These reactions are instinctive. They're hard-wired into our bodies and no amount of training will completely remove them. However, effective training methods can reduce the harmful aspects of these phenomena (such as auditory exclusion, denial, etc.) and improve the beneficial byproducts, such as tachypsychia (things seem to slow down to a manageable rate of speed). Training can also increase fine motor skill performance as the body learns to adapt to the "adrenaline dump" associated with a violent encounter.

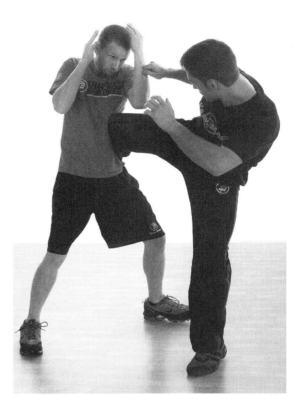

Training Methods to Improve Responses

Proper training drills acclimatize the practitioner to the physical and psychological stress of a violent encounter. Of course, no training drill can safely replicate the danger and stress of a real, life-threatening situation. However, we can create drills that simulate those sensations to a lesser degree or drills that create one or two aspects of stress. For instance, take tunnel vision and auditory exclusion. It's relatively easy to create drills that simulate stress, and then require students to deal with the immediate danger while also remaining aware of their surroundings.

Example 1: For this drill, you'll need three people (one defender and two attackers) as well as one training shield. The defender will need to know basic combatives, as well as at least one self-defense technique (say, for example, Choke from the Front, page 132). The defender stands in a neutral (unprepared) position with eyes closed. The attacker with the pad moves to a new position after the defender has closed his eyes. The empty-handed attacker attacks with a Choke from the Front. The defender must react efficiently and aggressively, while also scanning the room for the other attacker. Once that attacker approaches, the defender pushes away from the original attacker and deals with the new threat.

Note: Beginners will have a tendency to sacrifice the power and effectiveness of their counterattacks in order to watch for the second attacker. This is not allowed! The defender must learn to counterattack explosively to neutralize the first attacker and also be aware of the environment.

Example 2: To train away from auditory exclusion, we do many stress drills during which students must listen for a command, either from the instructor or from their partner. The action itself is incidental—it can be something as simple as turning and sprinting to the other end of the room and then coming back, or as complicated as listening for a specific set of movements such as a new punch combination, running to one of several new areas of the room, etc. It is the cognitive act of hearing and acknowledging, while still dealing with the immediate threat, that is vital.

Example 3: To acclimatize new students to the sensation of being hit and continuing to fight, we do simple drills wherein they must continually punch a pad while a third person slaps and strikes them. These strikes are light at first so that beginners don't shut down, but as the student becomes used to the contact, the power is increased to a manageable degree. It's not pleasant, but it's more desirable than being shocked by the sting of a blow during a real fight.

Again, none of these drills are the same as a real violent encounter, but they do simulate various aspects of a real fight. We've had law-enforcement officers tell us, during some of our more extreme drills, that the emotional reactions they experienced during our drills were the same as they experienced during firefights while on duty. The more they can train under these circumstances, the more effective they'll be during a real encounter. This sort of training will save their lives, or the lives of someone near them.

Visualization

As you undoubtedly know by now, you won't find anything "zen" in Krav Maga. We don't meditate, or find our center, or work on our *chi*. There's a place for such things in one's life, but you won't find that place inside a Krav Maga school.

There is, however, some value in the idea of visualization. Visualization is simply the act of playing out a scenario in your head. See it as clearly as you possibly can. Imagine every detail—not just the attacker's face, but his expression; not just the type of attack, but the angle of his arm, the size of his hands, etc. See yourself making the defense. You are, in effect, training your brain to tell your body to react with the appropriate defense based on the situation. We can't all spend every day at the training center. But using basic visualization techniques, you can double or triple your training time. Having trouble with a headlock defense? Visualize doing it correctly a hundred times. You'll find yourself improving your actual physical technique as well.

But there's more to visualization than just the improvement of physical movement. There's a psychological aspect as well. We fear what is unfamiliar to us. Visualizing violent encounters helps us to "know" them (at least a little) before they happen. We create the opportunity to reduce our fear of that critical moment by dealing with it in our minds first. Familiarity reduces stress. Reduced stress leads to shorter reaction time, which means we are ultimately training ourselves to react more aggressively and decisively to neutralize the threat.

We'll take this one step farther. We encourage you not only to visualize yourself making a successful technique. We'd like you to spend one or two moments visualizing failure. Imagine the worst-case scenario. Come to accept that it might happen. Lose your fear of it. Remember, we fear what we don't understand. Come to understand that no one is perfect, and that every one of us might fail under stress. Imagine failing in a technique. What would you do next? How would you react and recover?

Imagining failure does not mean quitting. It means preparing for reality. However, don't spend too much time imagining failure. You don't want to train your brain to make the wrong technique or to expect failure. The only purpose of this small aspect of training is to help remove the stress of failing. Once you've done a little of this worst-case scenario work, spend more of your time visualizing success: defending quickly and decisively, counterattacking powerfully, and neutralizing the assailant.

Example:

> *Imagine that it's night. You walk to your front door, holding a bag of groceries in your left hand. With your right hand, you reach into your pocket or purse for your keys. You hear a motion behind you, but before you can turn, you feel an arm wrap around your throat, putting you into a headlock. You're pulled backward, off balance. You feel intense pressure on the sides of your neck (your carotid arteries) and on your windpipe. You smell beer and cheap aftershave. You feel his shoulder and head pressed against the back of your head. You're aware of the attacker's hands clasped together, just over your left shoulder.*
>
> *You drop the bag of groceries. Your hands fly up, over your left shoulder, bent into hooks. They pluck explosively at the attacker's hands as you turn your left shoulder sharply into your attacker. The pluck and the turn have made a little space, and now you turn your chin. You slide your head out of the opening and continue turning. The groceries are scattered underfoot. The door is at your back and you're now facing the attacker. You deliver a knee to the attacker's groin. He's wearing a dark brown shirt and denim jeans. He doubles over, but as he does he tries to grab your legs. You brace your forearms against his shoulder, keep him away, and you deliver another knee, this time to his midsection. He grunts as the air is driven from his lungs. He drops to his knees, but you can still feel him leaning forward, grabbing for you. You deliver another knee, this time to his face. You see a shaved head, an unshaven face. You feel your knee smash into his nose. He drops to the ground.*
>
> *You step back and assess the situation. There are no other attackers. He's still on his stomach, coughing and sputtering. He appears to be in his mid-twenties, Caucasian. He has big hands. A tattoo on his neck looks like barbed wire. You keep your eyes on him and dig your keys out of your pocket or purse. Keep your eyes on him. Feel for the door and unlock it. Go inside. Lock the door. Go directly to the phone and dial 9-1-1. The phone is portable. Go back to the door. Look or listen for more activity from the attacker. Remember your address. Say it clearly and distinctly.*

This is a simple example, of course, but notice the detail. Train yourself to notice small details as they'll help in articulating the attack and in finding the attacker if he avoids arrest initially.

Although visualization will never take the place of actual training, we do believe that if you add some visualization exercises to your training, you'll see a marked improvement in both your techniques and your ability to deal with the stress of a violent encounter.

Use of Force

"Will I get in trouble with the law if I use self-defense?" This question inevitably arises during training. It's a valid and pertinent question. Unfortunately, there is no clean and simple answer because the rightness of your actions depends completely on the context.

Before we go any further, we should take a moment to make a distinction between a civil complaint and criminal charges. In our rather litigious society, it seems that anyone can bring a lawsuit against anyone else for almost anything. This isn't quite true—judges will usually throw out the obviously frivolous cases—but you

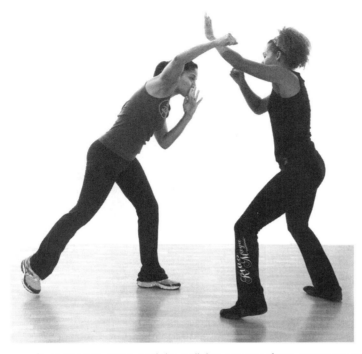

should begin your self-defense training knowing that, even if you're completely reasonable in your use of self-defense, and the police and district attorney agree with that conclusion, your assailant may try to file a civil suit against you. This doesn't mean the assailant will win the case, but it does mean you may have to hire legal representation to prove your point.

Criminal cases, on the other hand, tend to adhere to a higher standard. Police officers must collect evidence (and, indeed, decide whether or not to arrest any of the participants). A deputy district attorney must review that evidence to decide if a crime has been committed, and if there is enough evidence to take to trial. All agents of the law enforcement and justice system use their judgment, but they're guided by established and relatively predictable laws and policies. Unfortunately, those laws can vary from state to state, and the policies can vary from county to county. Additionally, this book will most likely be read by practitioners in countries other than the United States. It is beyond the scope of this book to describe every nuance of Use of Force law for every region and reader. We can, however, discuss general guidelines that will be familiar to most readers.

No Retribution

You are not allowed to hurt people simply because you think they deserve it. For instance, let's say someone attacks you and you defend yourself while delivering one kick to his groin. If that one kick incapacitates him, the law states that you no longer have a right to harm him. You cannot strike him two or three more times simply because you think he deserves it for attacking you. The law allows for self-defense (under conditions described below), but not retribution. Assuming the context is appropriate, you're allowed to do enough to keep yourself safe, and no more.

Reasonable Man Standard

We often hear people say that, after using self-defense, they'll just tell the police, "I was in fear for my life." This is appropriate (assuming it's true), but not sufficient. In the end, what you felt is not the only factor because, for all society knows, you might be a paranoid schizophrenic who is always in fear for your life. In the United States, the standard to which you will be held is somewhat higher, and can be stated this way:

You are allowed to use whatever force a reasonable person, in your situation, would feel is necessary to protect himself.

The key word, of course, is "reasonable." This inserts a level of objectivity to the situation. If a 6'5" man walks up to a small woman in a darkened parking lot and grabs her by the throat, a reasonable person in her situation would feel extremely threatened and respond with very aggressive self-defense to remain safe. If, however, the 5' woman attacks the much larger man, a reasonable person might assume that the man might need a lower level of force to protect himself from the woman. *Note:* This does *not* mean he isn't allowed to defend himself; it just means that he might be expected to use more restraint.

The devil is in the details, of course, and those details may influence the reasonable person's opinion. For instance, if the female attacker is a highly trained martial artist and the man has a broken leg, we might reasonably assume a slightly different standard. Assuming he is the attacker, we might expect her to defend herself, disengage, and retreat, rather than smashing his head repeatedly into the ground. There is a point at which the use of force begins to seem like excessive force and, in such a situation, the woman would have to explain why she felt the need to treat the attacker's head like a basketball.

The police and the district attorney's office will use the Reasonable Man standard (or some standard very similar to this) and take into account any specifics that might clearly create the context in their decision to file criminal charges. Use of Force standards for law enforcement officers vary slightly, due to the nature of their jobs. Generally speaking, law enforcement officers are allowed to use one level of force higher than is being used against them so that they can control the situation and arrest the suspect. Civilians are not tasked with the responsibility to arrest offenders. Therefore, in many regions there is no authority to use a higher level of force. Rather, as stated above, civilians are permitted to use enough force to defend themselves…and, of course, the definition of "enough force" falls back to the Reasonable Man standard. Depending on the situation, "enough force" might mean one kick to the groin, but it might also mean picking up a rock and beating your assailant until he is incapacitated.

This last part is, in the end, the message Krav Maga delivers to its students. Use no more force than is necessary…but be totally willing and committed to use whatever force is needed to keep you safe!

Women and Self-Defense

Many women fear that they will be victims of a violent and/or sexual assault. Tragically, this fear has its foundation in fact. According to the Rape, Abuse & Incest National Network, one out of every six American women has been the victim of an attempted or completed rape in her lifetime. Often, women are physically and/or sexually abused by someone they know.

Society has a responsibility to change itself so that women are not put at risk. However, until that happens, women should make every reasonable effort to make themselves safer. Women need to learn to defend themselves, regardless of age or ability. Fortunately, Krav Maga is already designed for women's self-defense needs.

Statistics from several major studies done in the last 20 years show that women who fight back increase their chances of avoiding rape. In 1985, Pauline Bart and Patricia O'Brien published a study called "Stopping Rape: Successful Survival Strategies." In 1993, Sarah Ullman and Raymond Knight published a study called "The Efficacy of Women's Resistance Strategies in Rape Situations." Another article that bears mention was published in 1999 by S. Margaret Heyden, Billie Francis Anger, Tiel Theng-Woo Jackson, and Todd David Ellner. The article, titled "Fighting Back Works: The Case for Advocating and Teaching Self-Defense against Rape," summarizes the results of multiple studies (including the Bart & O'Brien work mentioned above) and offers an interesting breakdown of various types of resistance. All these publications are, in our opinion, recommended reading for anyone interested in detailed statistical analysis of rape situations and various types of resistance used by women.

The conclusion: Approximately 70 percent of women who fight back during an assault avoid rape. The actual percentage varies from study to study, but the vast majority of studies indicate that some level of active resistance improves a woman's chances of avoiding rape.

"Fighting Back Works" creates categories of resistance that prove useful to our discussion. Resistance can be classified in the following ways:

- Non-forceful verbal resistance (crying, pleading, reasoning, etc.)
- Forceful verbal resistance (yelling and screaming)
- Non-forceful physical resistance (running)
- Forceful physical resistance (fighting back)

The results of several studies report that reactions such as crying or reasoning are least likely to work. In one study, women who tried these strategies avoided rape only 4 percent of the time. In cases where women offered forceful verbal resistance, they successfully avoided rape 50 to 56 percent of the time. The data on non-forceful physical resistance (running) was mixed, with the results ranging widely. One study suggested that running worked 55 percent of the time, but the Bart and O'Brien study reported that 85 percent of the women who ran successfully avoided rape. As for the women who fought back forcefully, they avoided rape anywhere from 55 to 86 percent of the time.

There are a lot of numbers listed here, and we should not forget that each of these "percentages" is a living, breathing human being who was put in a horrible situation. But the studies give us valuable information: Fighting back increases your chances of avoiding rape.

Of course, there are no guarantees. Even if the 70 percent number quoted above holds true, that still means that 30 percent of women who actively fight back are still raped. There is no silver lining in that dark cloud, but there is one more important statistic: Studies indicate that women who fight back are no more likely to suffer additional physical violence (such as additional beatings or abuse) than women who do not.

The bottom line is clear: You have nothing to lose by fighting back, and everything to gain.

Fighting Back

Assuming that these studies are correct, how do women learn to fight back? Krav Maga is a system designed for use by men and women, and the instinct-based foundations of the techniques mean they can be accessed during the stress of a rape attempt.

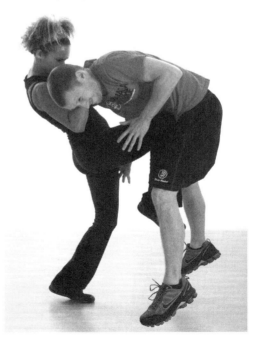

The acknowledgement of your instinctive reactions under stress is important. For example, Krav Maga offers a technique for when the attacker is on top of you and "in your guard" (between your legs). In other systems such as Brazilian jiu-jitsu (and, indeed, later in Krav Maga), you would learn very effective techniques for wrapping your legs around an attacker, controlling him from beneath, and then reversing or submitting him. These techniques are proven to be effective. *However*, they're not instinctive. Telling a woman who is about to be raped that she should wrap her legs around her attacker goes against every instinct she is feeling in that moment. This is why, for beginners, we teach the Kicking Off from the Guard technique (see page 169). It's an effective version of the defender's instinct to keep the attacker away.

What does a rapist look like?

There is no specific demographic for rapists, except that they're overwhelmingly male. Rapists come in all shapes and sizes, nationalities, and ethnicities. They do not have a particular "look." The truth is that the majority of rape victims are attacked by assailants they know (in one 2000 study done by the American Medical Association, 80 percent of the attackers were friends, acquaintances, intimates, or family members).

Also, Krav Maga's emphasis on "no rules" fighting is an important one for women. If you decide to fight back, you should fight as though your life is on the line. Pull out every tool you have, and put away every inhibition that will stop you from using them. Go for vulnerable targets such as the groin, eyes, and throat. If you cannot reach these areas, gouge skin (the face is best, but tear away at any sensitive area you can reach, such as the sides, thighs, and ears). Bite. Yes, we know there are valid concerns about the transfer of bodily fluids, but you must deal with the immediate danger first. Your teeth and jaw are valuable weapons, and you use them every day to crunch objects much harder than human flesh. Use them to defend yourself!

Don't look like a victim

Don't appear to be a victim. Walk confidently, and remain aware of your surroundings. Rapists are predators, and predators by nature look for the easiest prey they can find. This is no guarantee of avoiding an assault, however. While writing this chapter, one of the authors had to counsel a female student who was groped (not raped) by a man passing her on the street. She handled herself well, but was startled to have been "chosen" because she carries herself with confidence and does not look like a victim.

Remember, any kind of sexual assault is NOT the fault of the victim. A woman who is attacked is not responsible for an assailant's actions if she doesn't look like a female mixed martial arts champion. He is at fault for assaulting the woman. Carrying yourself with confidence and remaining aware of your surroundings will not decrease your chances of being attacked to zero, but it will turn the odds in your favor.

Trust your instincts

If a person or situation gives you a bad feeling, listen to that feeling. Leave the person, leave the situation, leave the area. Most people (and women more than men) are socially conditioned to avoid embarrassing or insulting other people.

Let's ask this question: Imagine you step onto a lonely elevator at night. The elevator moves one floor, and when the door opens, a man walks in. Immediately, you feel uncomfortable. You're not sure why, but something about him puts you on edge. What would you do?

The safest thing to do is to exit the elevator immediately, even if that means pushing through the door before it closes, or immediately pushing the button for the next floor and getting off.

Most people will avoid doing this because it publicly displays your opinion of the stranger. It's potentially insulting to him, and we're taught to avoid intentionally insulting strangers in public situations.

But so what? We need to be more concerned about our own safety than the potential insult to a stranger. We're not harming him in any way. No real damage is done. But if we stay on the elevator, and it turns out our instincts were correct, then we have put ourselves in danger.

Listen to your instincts. Make trusting your instincts more important than a stranger's opinion of you.

Stranger behavior

In the scenario above, we included no clues as to why the man put us on edge. We just had an instinctive feeling. He made us uncomfortable. But often, in the moments that precede assaults, there are indicators: men who strike up and then pursue an obviously unwanted conversation; men who stand too close; men who stare.

Whole books have been dedicated to topics like this (one that we highly recommend is Gavin de Becker's *The Gift of Fear*). It is beyond this book's capacity to go into great detail about these sorts of behavior. We can, however, summarize the topic into one simple, absolute, and understandable concept:

Men who mean you no harm go out of their way not *to make you uncomfortable.*

A socially attuned man getting in the elevator with you will automatically stand as far from you as possible, and make himself as unobtrusive as he can. A man walking behind you on a lonely sidewalk will almost always slow down, or alter course so that he is not directly at your back. A man passing you in a darkened parking lot on the way to his car will shy away from you, giving you space, as if to indicate that he is definitely not coming your way.

We all do these things without giving them much thought because we are operating under the same social contract together. Rapists and other attackers are not. They are either unaware of the discomfort they cause, or they enjoy it. The moment a man shows willingness to make you uncomfortable, he is telling you that his intentions are not normal. We can't say for sure that he's a rapist or that he's going to assault you (for all we know, he may be an insurance salesman desperate to make one final sale), but he has some sort of intention toward you, and you are right to be on your guard.

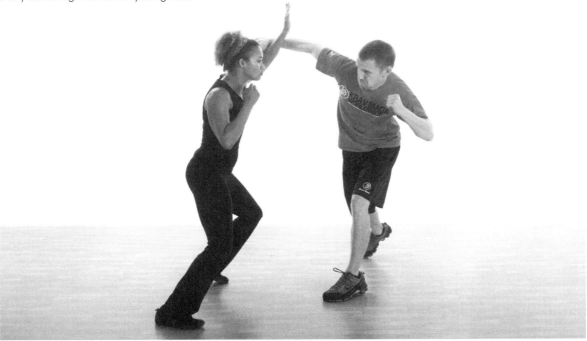

Physical training

All the techniques in this book work. All of them have been performed on the street, under stress, by someone just like you. But techniques are worthless if you don't apply them aggressively and decisively, determined to do whatever it takes to drive off your attacker. Although we encourage you to learn the actual techniques in this book and train yourself to apply them cleanly under stress, the truth is that developing a strong fighting spirit is more important. Fighting spirit without technique does some good. Technique without fighting spirit is meaningless.

Put yourself through some of the drills mentioned in this book, or find a local Krav Maga school (if one isn't available, try any school that teaches real, practical, reality-based self-defense) and go through stress drills.

If you think you're not the aggressive type, you're wrong. We can say that without even meeting you. Everyone has some aggressiveness in them. Maybe you can't rouse yourself to defend yourself. Then imagine your daughter, son, or mother being attacked. Imagine what might happen to someone you love if you do not stop the assailant. Fight for yourself. Fight for someone else. But whatever you do, fight.

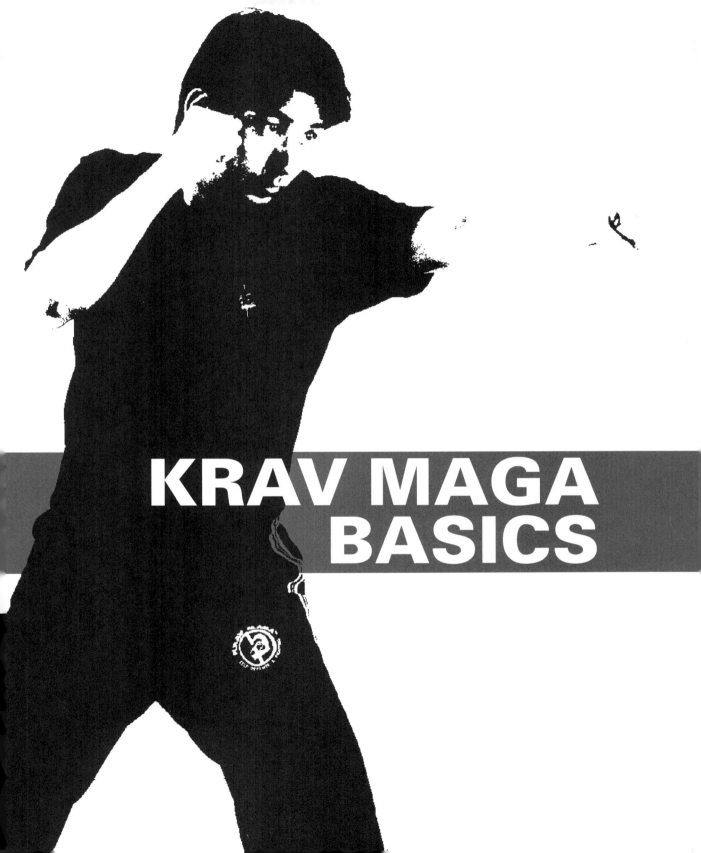

KRAV MAGA
BASICS

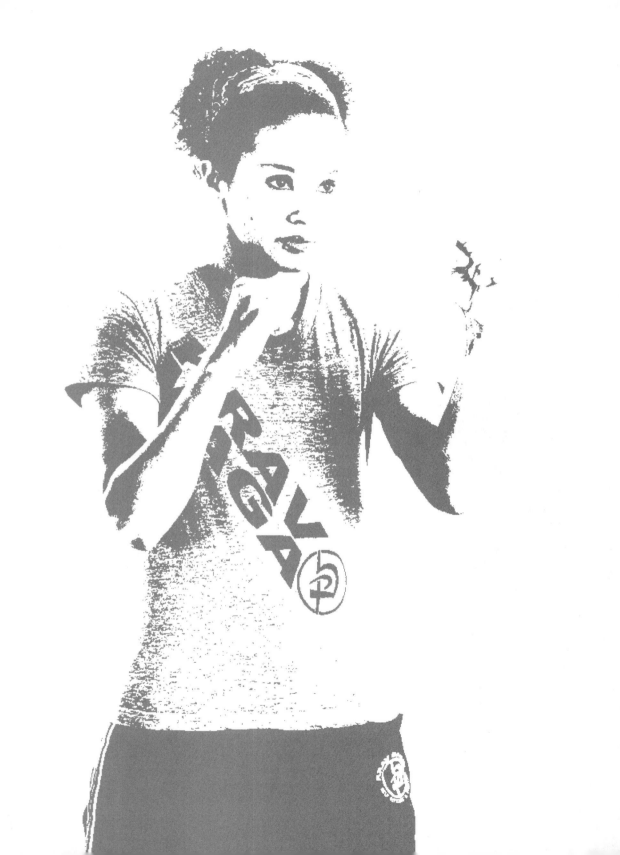

Warm-Up Overview

Before you can begin studying Krav Maga, you must prepare your body for the work at hand. We'd like you to keep in mind two of the most basic Krav Maga principles.

Krav Maga Principle #1: *Go home safe.* This principle applies equally to your workout and training in Krav Maga as it does to surviving a violent street confrontation—so warm up and go home safe.

Krav Maga Principle #2: *Safety in training.* When we train in Krav Maga, we train with realistic scenarios and intensity. If your body is not prepared for the demand you place on it or you have an unsafe training environment, you may get injured, which violates Krav Maga Principle #1. We do not violate principles, so warmeth thyself up!

This section incorporates three different warm-up methods: shadowboxing, joint mobilization, and preparation movements.

1. Shadowboxing

The first goal of this warm-up is to elevate your core body temperature and prepare you physically and mentally for training. The increased core temperature will decrease your risk of injury and improve your performance. Fighting is dynamic and requires the ability to move your body from point A to B. Accordingly, your warm-up must be dynamic as well.

Shadowboxing is one of the best ways to warm up the body and simultaneously work on movement, a necessary fighting skill. It also hones dynamic stability/balance and muscular coordination/strength. When you move in a fighting stance, you must keep a balance between your ability to move quickly and your stability for counterattacks. The goal is to maintain a proper stance each and every time you move your feet. This takes practice, which is why we use basic shadowboxing and movement as a warm-up. Start with a leisurely pace and slowly add techniques, speed, and movement to increase the difficulty. Please refer to page 64 for detailed description of basic stances and movement.

2. Joint Mobilization

This warm-up will also increase the dynamic flexibility and range of motion of your joints and muscles, preparing your body for the upcoming Krav Maga techniques. By using exercises and movement patterns that mimic the movements in Krav Maga, you receive all the benefits of a traditional warm-up with the added benefit of repetition of basic movement patterns.

3. Preparation Movements

The preparation movements are designed to increase dynamic flexibility and increase balance/stability while preparing the body for movement. These movements can be done in place or with a step in between to allow for movement. Each exercise should be done for 5 repetitions per side.

Basic Shadowboxing with Weight Shift

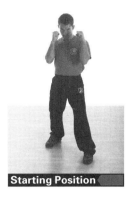

Starting Position

Starting Position: Basic left-leg-forward fighting stance.

1-2 Slowly shift your weight from the front foot to the back foot, keeping your feet in place. Do this for 30 seconds.

3-4 Now shift your weight left to right and right to left in a side-to-side fashion. Do this for 30 seconds.

Now combine the two movements, shifting your weight forward, back, left, and right, mixing up the order of the weight shift. Do this for 1 minute.

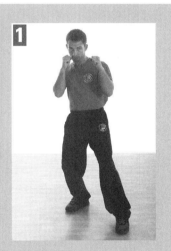

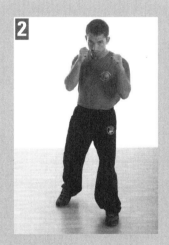

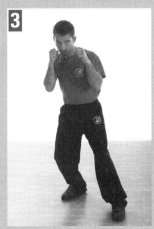

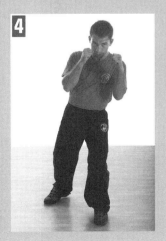

Basic Shadowboxing with Movement

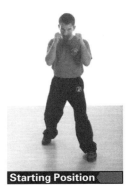

Starting Position

Starting Position: Basic left-leg-forward fighting stance.

1 Keeping your chin down and hands up, shift your weight to your back foot and step the front foot forward, opening the stance.

2 Close the stance by moving your rear foot forward the same distance.

3 Shift your weight to your right foot and step to the left with your left foot.

4 Close the stance by moving your right foot to the left the same distance.

5 Shift your weight to your left foot and step to the right with your right foot.

6 Close the stance by moving your left foot to the right the same distance.

Continue to move forward and back, then left to right and right to left, for 2 minutes. Relax, breathe, and find your balance.

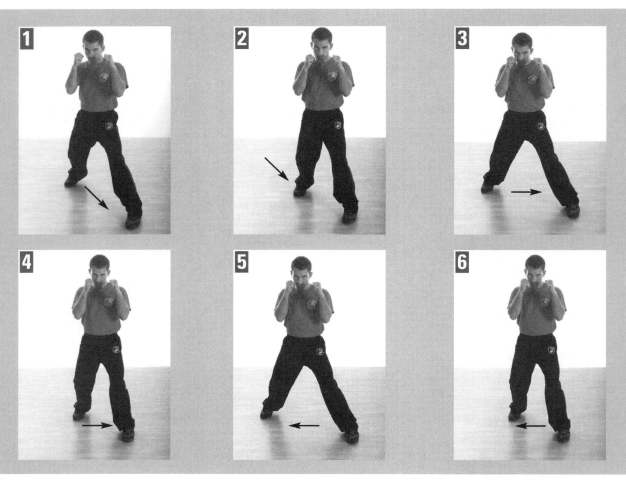

Neck Rotation

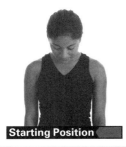

Starting Position

Starting Position: Stand with your feet hip-width apart and bing your chin to your chest.

1 Slowly roll your head in a half circle to the right.

2 Slowly roll your head in a half circle to the left.

Repeat several times.

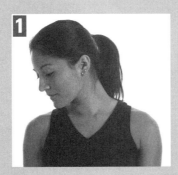

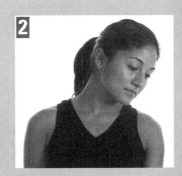

Shoulder Rotation

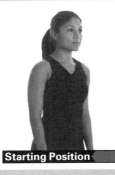

Starting Position

Starting Position: Stand with proper alignment.

1 Bring your shoulders to your ears.

2 Roll them forward and down to the starting position.

Continue rolling them in a circle back up. Repeat several times.

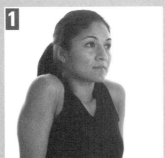

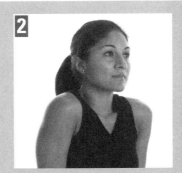

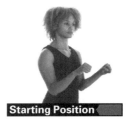

Starting Position (label)

Starting Position: Stand with proper alignment.

1 Circle your wrists clockwise.

2 Circle your wrists counterclockwise.

Repeat several times.

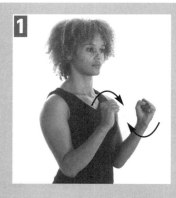
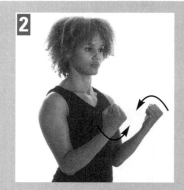

Hip Rotation

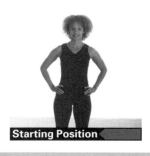

Starting Position (label)

Starting Position: Stand with your feet about hip-width apart and place your hands on your hips.

1 Circle your hips in a clockwise direction.

2 Circle your hips in a counterclockwise direction.

Repeat both directions several times.

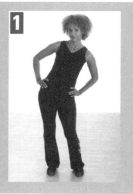
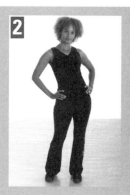

Torso Rotation

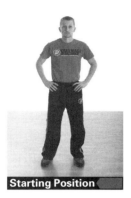

Starting Position (image label)

Starting Position: Stand with your feet about hip-width apart, place your hands on your hips, and slightly bend your knees.

1 Start the rotation by bending to your right side, taking your right elbow toward the floor.

2 Slowly bend your body forward and down toward the center, keeping your head forward.

3 Continue circling your torso to a left side bend.

4 Circle back to center, taking care not to extend your back.

Repeat to the right and left several times.

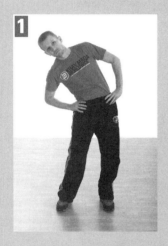

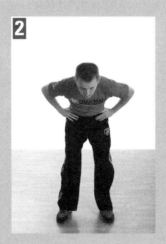

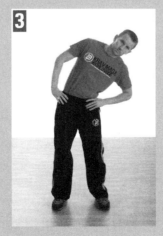

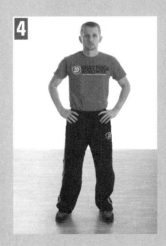

Knee Rotation

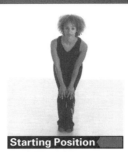

Starting Position

Starting Position: Stand with your feet together, bend your knees slightly, and place your hands on your knees.

1 Circle your knees in a clockwise direction.

2 Circle your knees in a counter-clockwise direction.

Repeat both directions several times.

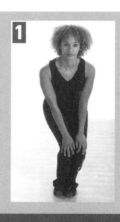

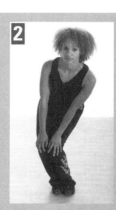

Ankle Rotation

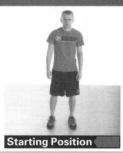

Starting Position

Starting Position: Stand with your feet about hip-width apart.

1 Raise your right knee to hip height and circle your ankle in a clock-wise direction.

2 Keeping your knee raised, circle your ankle in a counterclockwise direction.

Repeat on the other leg, and then repeat several times on both legs.

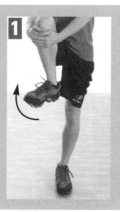

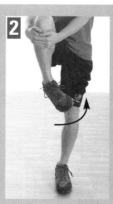

High Knees

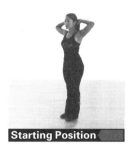

Starting Position

Starting Position: Stand with your feet about hip-width apart and place your hands behind your head.

1 Raise your right knee to hip height, pulling your toes up.

You should have 90-degree bends at the hip, knee, and ankle. Balance for one beat.

Perform on the left side. Repeat 4 times on each side.

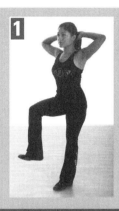

High Knees with Rotation

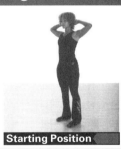

Starting Position

Starting Position: Stand with your feet about hip-width apart and place your hands behind your head.

1 Raise your left knee to hip height, pull your toes up, and rotate your

right elbow to your right knee. Balance for one beat.

Perform on the other side. Repeat 4 times on each side.

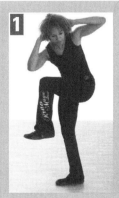

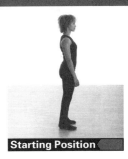

Starting Position

Starting Position: Stand with your feet about hip-width apart.

1 Maintaining an upright posture and keeping your bellybutton in, grab your right ankle with your right hand and pull your heel toward your rear end.

Perform on the other side. Repeat 4 times on each side.

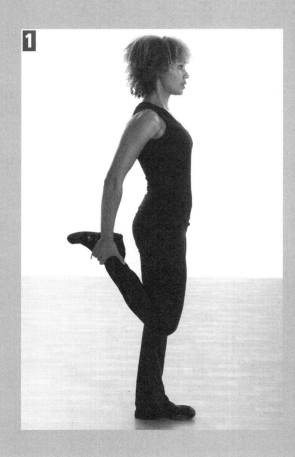

Defensive Front Kick (Balance/Stretch)

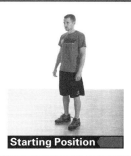

Starting Position

Starting Position: Stand with your feet about hip-width apart.

1 Raise your knee to hip height.

2 Extend your leg and flex your toes toward you. Hold for one beat.

Bring your knee back in before returning to starting position. Perform on the other side. Repeat 4 times on each side.

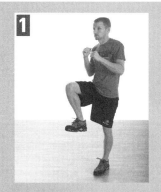
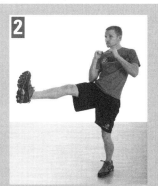

Tip: Exhale and pull your bellybutton slightly in. This will help you to maintain proper alignment in your spine and pelvis.

Defensive Front Kick (Swing)

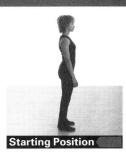

Starting Position

Maintain the alignment of your spine and pelvis while gradually increasing the swing of the leg up and down, each time working for more height.

Starting Position: Stand with your feet about hip-width apart.

1 Exhale and pull in your bellybutton to remain tall; lift your left leg as high as possible.

Slowly return to starting position and perform on the other side. Repeat 4 times on each side.

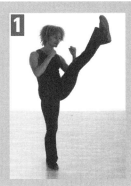

Back Kick (Hinge Over)

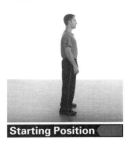

Starting Position

Starting Position: Stand with your feet about hip-width apart.

1 Keeping a long spine, raise your right heel up and hinge your upper body forward toward the floor. Allow your rising leg to counterbalance your upper body. Extend your leg until your heel reaches waist height. Hold for one beat.

Return to starting position and perform on the other side. Repeat 4 times on each side.

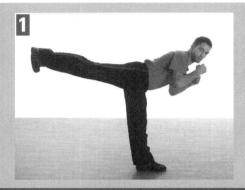

Back Kick (Swing)

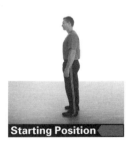

Starting Position

The goal of this exercise is to maintain the alignment of your spine and pelvis while gradually increasing the swing of the leg.

Starting Position: Stand with your feet about hip-width apart.

1 Keeping a long spine, drive your left heel up and lean your upper body toward the floor. Your leg should make a swinging motion, stopping before the heel of your foot begins to move close to your body.

Return to starting position and perform on the other side. Repeat 4 times on each side.

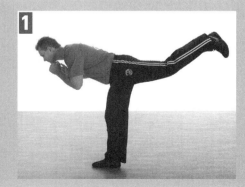

Penetration Lunge (Stretch)

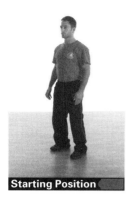

Starting Position

Starting Position: Stand with your feet about hip-width apart.

1 Take a long step forward with your right foot, sinking down until your knee reaches a 90-degree bend.

2 Push off the front leg to return to starting position. Your upper body can hinge forward slightly at the waist as long as your spine remains long.

Perform on the other side. Repeat 4 times on each side.

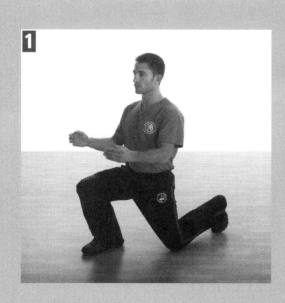

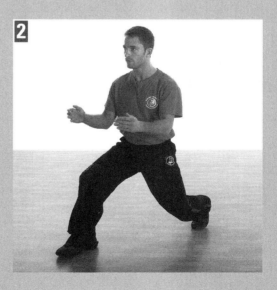

Penetration Lunge with Upper Body Rotation

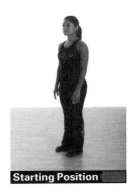

Starting Position

Starting Position: Stand with your feet about hip-width apart.

1 Raise your arms, interlock your fingers with the index fingers extended (think *Charlie's Angels*), and take a long step forward with your left leg, sinking down until your front knee reaches a 90-degree bend.

2 As you reach the end of the lunge, rotate your upper body like a turret toward your left side.

Return your upper body to center before pushing off the front leg to return to starting position. Perform on the other side. Repeat 4 times on each side.

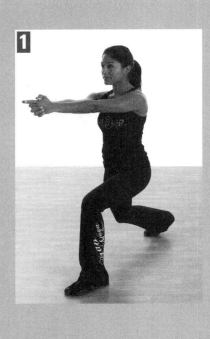

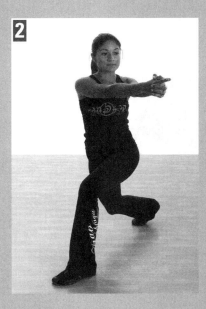

Side Lunge to Balance

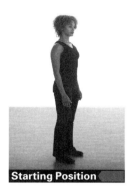

Starting Position

Starting Position: Stand with your feet about hip-width apart.

1 Take a long step with your left leg to your left side and sink down until the knee reaches 90 degrees. Hold for one beat here. Maintain a long spine; it's normal to have to sit back a bit to maintain balance.

2 For the second part of this exercise, drive off the right leg, pushing up to a standing balance position on the left leg.

3 Pull the right leg up to waist height, with the knee and ankle bent at 90 degrees.

Hold a beat and set the foot down. Repeat on the other side.

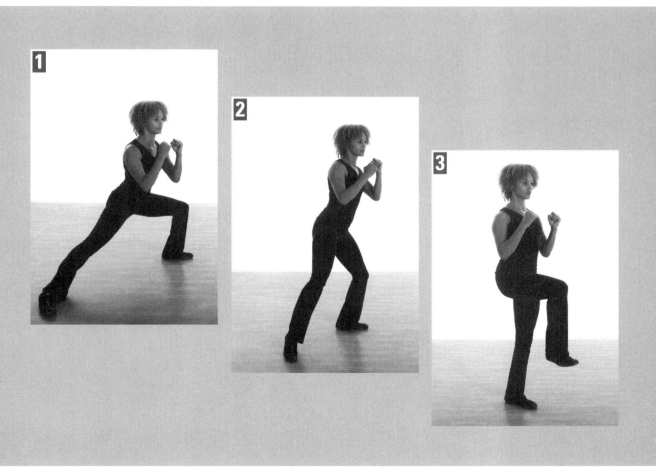

This exercise features three moves. The goal is to move slowly, at least 6 beats per section. Slowly work your way through this combo, feeling the stretch in each section. Start with 5 total repetitions.

Slow Takedown Defense

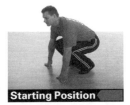

Starting Position

Starting Position: Squat down, keeping your head up, and place your hands on the floor in front of your feet with your fingers facing out.

1 Jump your feet back.

2 Slowly allow your waist to sink to the floor and look up, keeping your shoulders back and down.

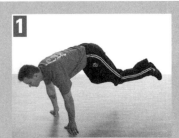

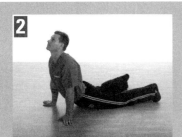

Bull Post

If you practice yoga, you'll recognize this as Downward-facing Dog.

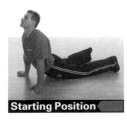

Starting Position

Starting Position: The bottom of the takedown defense.

1 Shift your hips up and back, turn your fingers forward, and spread your fingers wide. Press into the floor as you drive your shoulders away from your ears. Push your hips up and back while pressing your hands into the floor. Pull your chest toward your thighs and glide your hips back (as in downward-facing dog position). Take a beat here to feel the stretch. Maintain a long spine from your tailbone to the top of your head.

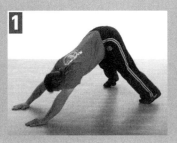

Caterpillar

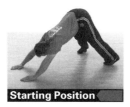
Starting Position

Starting Position: The extended Bull Post.

1 Baby-step your hands back toward your feet while feeling the stretch in the backs of your legs and calves.

2-3 Once you've reached your stretch limit, slightly bend your knees and slowly rise up one bit at a time to a standing position

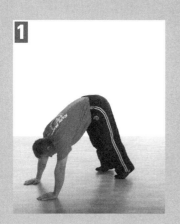

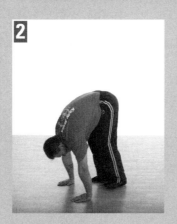

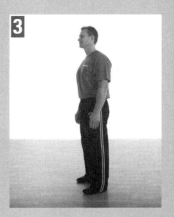

Conditioning for Krav Maga

The muscular and cardiovascular conditioning program Krav-FIT is designed to develop a beginning student's overall fitness level as well as provide "hidden repetition" on basic movement patterns that are necessary for training for the fight. A normal workout will involve the following: warm-up (10 to 15 minutes), alignment postures (5 minutes), circuit training (such as Krav-FIT workout; 15 to 25 minutes), and cool-down with alignment postures and a focus on controlling your breathing.

Before starting your daily training in Krav Maga, it's important to give the body a reference point for muscle length and alignment. The alignment postures, when done correctly, do just that and have the added benefit of correcting common spinal misalignments. We recommend that you do the alignment postures in front of a mirror for visual feedback. This will help you recognize misalignments or collapsing of the spine.

The muscular conditioning program aims to develop strength and muscular endurance that's vital to your progress in Krav Maga training. It's important to use proper form to avoid injury, so be sure to read the instructions carefully. To work out at home, it's recommended that you purchase exercise tubing, an exercise mat, and a Jungle Gym (the latter is available at www.monkeybargym.com). A stop watch may also come in handy.

This program can be done as a supplement to your Krav Maga skills training or on opposite days depending on time and energy level. Warriors have been doing this type of muscular (bodyweight) conditioning for centuries—it's time to wake up your warrior and get Krav-FIT.

Krav-FIT Workout Challenge

Here is the basic Krav-FIT (Function Interval Training) workout, which should only be done once you've warmed up with the Krav Maga Warm-Up (see pages 37–53). Start with Level 1. Your goal is to always perform the prescribed number of repetitions with correct form, completing the entire circuit before resting. If you're just starting out, it's ok to rest as needed. Otherwise, try to keep moving. Once you've done Level 1 for a few weeks and need more of a challenge, progress to Level 2.

Follow these simple guidelines: 1) *Krav-FIT Rule #1: Clean what you catch.* In other words, finish what you start. If, for example, you start at Level 3 with 20 reps per exercise, you keep that number of reps for the complete circuit. 2) *Circuit–Repeat as Fast as Possible (AFAP).*

EXERCISE	page	LEVEL 1 *8 reps x 2 circuits*	LEVEL 2 *12 reps x 3 circuits*	LEVEL 3 *20 reps x 4 circuits*
Shadowboxing	62	2-min round	3-min round	5-min round
Sprawl	61			
Push-Up	59			
Shoulder Press	58			
Body Row	59	60 degrees	90 degrees	90 degrees
Squat	60			
Biceps Curl	58			
Top of Push-Up	57			
Bridge	57	30-sec hold	1-min hold	2-min hold
Plank	60	30-sec hold	1-min hold	2-min hold
Jump Rope	62	50 forward/50 backward	100/100	150/150

The Position: Stand tall with your feet shoulder-width apart. Point your feet straight ahead and place your weight evenly on both feet, front to back and side to side. Soften your knees and work your shins slightly forward. Keep your hands open wide and reach down toward your knees with your palms facing forward.

Open your chest and lengthen your entire spine. Think open and extend.

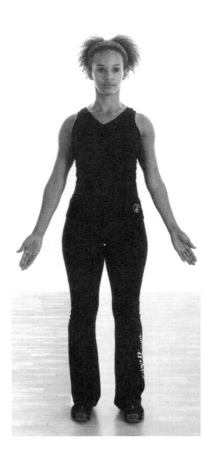
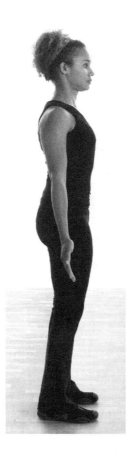

Bridge

target: hip, leg, and shoulder alignment

The Position: Lie on your back with your knees bent and your feet close to your butt. Place your arms down by your sides. Press your feet and the backs of your arms evenly into the floor, causing your butt to lift. Open your chest, push your shins slightly forward, and hold the bridge.

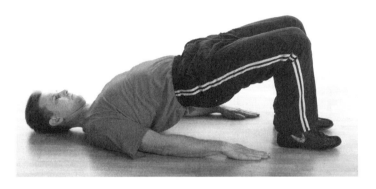

Top of Push-Up

target: shoulder, neck, back, and hip alignment

The Position: Get in a push-up position, placing your hands directly under your shoulders, extending your legs behind you, and balancing on the balls of your feet. Place even pressure in the palms of each hand and extend your fingers. Your elbows should be extended but not locked, and the insides of your elbows should face each other. Extend your spine from the tailbone to the top of your head; do not allow your upper or lower back to sag. Your spine should be in alignment from the top of your head to your heels.

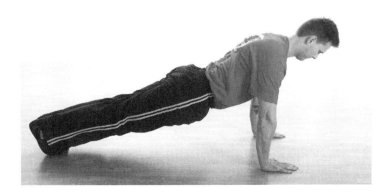

Shoulder Press

target: shoulders

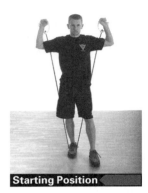

Starting Position

Starting Position: Assume Standing Alignment posture (page 56). Step on the band with one foot, making sure it sits in your arch. Clean the band to your shoulders.

1 Keeping your midsection tight, your chest lifted, and your shoulders down, extend your arms

overhead. Keep your knees soft and your shins forward with your weight even on both feet. Take care not to bend backward, which puts stress on the low back.

Return to starting position.

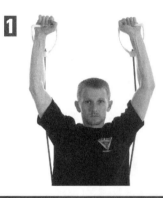

Biceps Curl

target: biceps

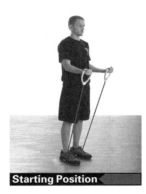

Starting Position

Starting Position: Assume Standing Alignment posture (page 56). Step on the band with both feet, making sure it sits in your arches. Keeping your elbows in, bring the band to waist height; your forearms should be parallel to the floor.

1 Keeping your shoulders/elbows stabilized and your midsection tight, curl the band up and in to your chest. Keep your knees soft, your shins forward, and your weight even on both feet.

Return to starting position.

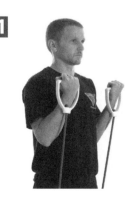

Push-Up

target: chest

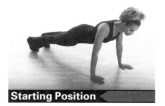

Starting Position

Starting Position: Assume Top of Push-Up alignment position (page 57).

1 Lower your body, touching your chest and hips to the ground at the same time.

2 Push back up to the starting position. Resist collapsing your spine or throwing your head forward. Maintain alignment (heels to top of head) by lifting your spine at the base of your neck so your head isn't hanging.

1
2

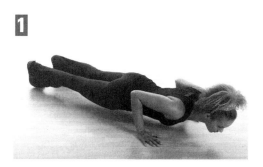

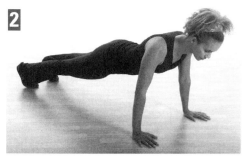

Body Row

target: back, arms

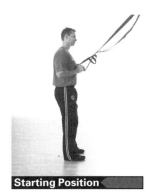

Starting Position

Starting Position: Place the Jungle Gym in a door with the door attachment. Hold the handles and take 4 steps back and measure the handles to your hips.

1 Lean your body back to 60 degrees with your arms straight and feet flat on the floor.

2 Pull your body upwards until your hands touch the outsides of your chest. Use your legs to assist the movement as needed.

Return to starting position.

Once this becomes easy, you can try leaning back 90 degrees.

1
2

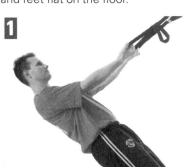

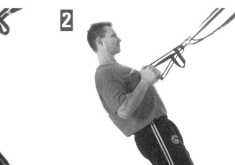

Plank

The Position: Assume Top of Push-Up alignment position (page 57), then lower down to your elbows. Maintain correct alignment from your heels to the top of head. Hold the position, lifting your spine from the base of your neck so your head doesn't hang.

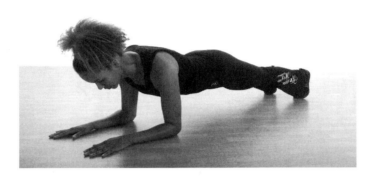

Squat

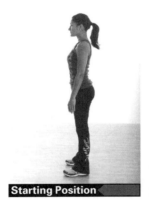

Starting Position

Starting Position: Assume Standing Alignment posture (page 56).

1 Keeping your chest forward and open, sit your butt back and down toward your heels, going as low as you can while maintaining alignment. Keep your weight even on both feet.

Return to standing.

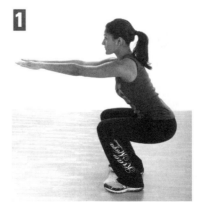

1

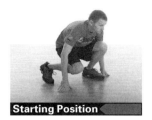

Starting Position

Starting Position: Squat down and place your hands on the floor just to the outsides of your feet. Your fingers should face out.

1 Jump your feet back to the incline posture position and drop your hips to the floor.

2 Spring up to fighting stance.

1

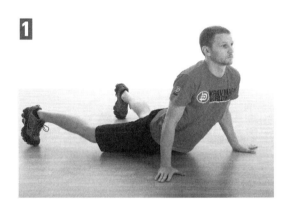

2

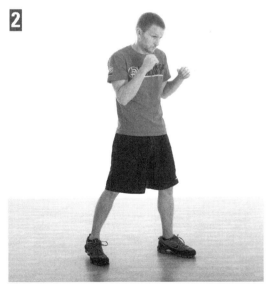

See pages 39–40 for step-by-step instructions. Once you get the hang of moving forward, backward, and side to side, add in straight punches, Inside Defense, 360° Defense. Keep moving, maintaining proper footwork—it helps to imagine fighting off an attacker, defending and counterattacking. Finally, add kicks, knees, and takedown defenses (sprawl).

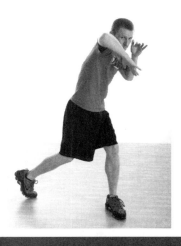

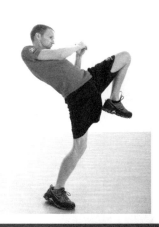

Jump Rope

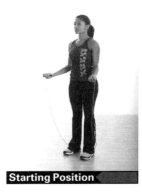

Starting Position

Starting Position: Assume Standing Alignment posture (page 56).

1 Jump rope forward and backward with single revolutions between jumps. Control your jump by jumping just enough to get the rope under your feet. Land as quietly as possible.

If you've never jumped rope before, begin with the X-Drill (page 63). This drill subscribes to the notion that if you can't perform an exercise, take it back a step and break down the movements to their basic elements. Perform the basic movements until you can do them easily and then progress up.

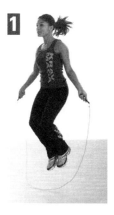

Starting Position: Begin by placing two jump ropes on the floor in an "X." Stand in one part of the X, close to the center.

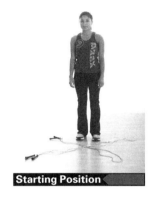

Starting Position

1-2 Squat down to a quarter-down position with your heels off the ground and then jump with both feet over the rope, just enough to miss the rope. Progress to both feet jumping forward and back over the rope, then try jumping both feet right into the next section and back. Finally, go crazy and jump from quadrant to quadrant.

Now keep time, building up to one minute of continuous jumping. Stage one complete—go buy a jump rope.

1

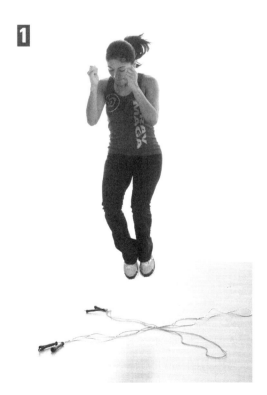

2

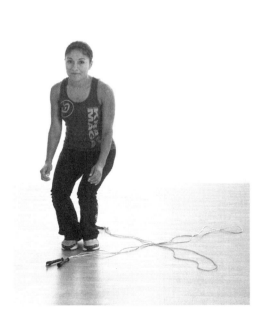

Training Positions

Krav Maga is a street fighting system. Most often, violent attacks occur when the defender is taken by surprise and is not ready or able to assume a "fighting" stance. Therefore, students of Krav Maga must learn to defend from many different positions, including when they have a very low state of readiness, and to respond to danger even from a neutral position. In basic Krav Maga training, emphasis is placed on three primary training positions. These basic elements are the tools you'll use to create effective and efficient reactions to a violent encounter. They are literally the foundation of each technique.

Neutral Position. Most self-defense in Krav Maga is trained from a position of disadvantage, commonly referred to as neutral position. This position is actually the absence of a stance. It's your natural, unprepared position, and it's a major component of Krav Maga training. Training from the neutral position allows the student to perform techniques when "late" or caught off guard.

The Stance: Stand with your feet about hip-width apart (or less), with your arms hanging to the sides.

Fighting Stance. The fighting stance in Krav Maga is used when preparing for a confrontation or after the initial attack and defense. The following description assumes a right-handed student. Left-handed students will simply substitute "right" for "left."

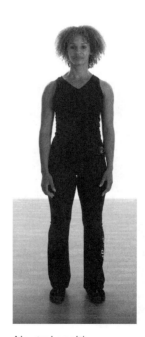

Neutral position

The Stance: Stand with your feet hip-width apart and take a comfortable step forward with your left foot. Keep your weight on the balls (not the heels) of your feet. The toes of both feet should generally point forward, but the forward foot may turn slightly inward for better balance.

Keeping your hands relaxed (not in fists), hold them up about chin height and a comfortable distance away from your face. Make sure your elbows are in and fairly close to your body, and your shoulders are relatively squared (not turned sideways) to an opponent. Keeping a constantly tight fist tightens up the muscles of the forearm and slows down reaction time. Tighten your fist as you send a punch; otherwise, keep your fingers more relaxed.

Groundfighting Position. When training on the ground, it's imperative to protect your head and tailbone from the ground, while keeping your feet between you and your attacker. There are various valid positions or "stances" while on the ground, but the back position is preferred at beginner levels. For more information on basic groundfighting, see pages 157–85.

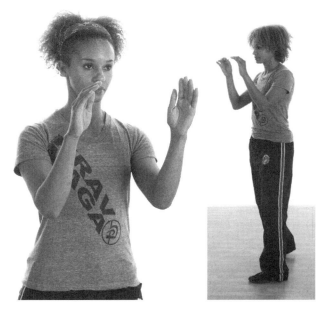

Fighting stances

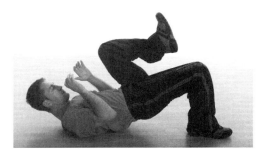

Groundfighting position

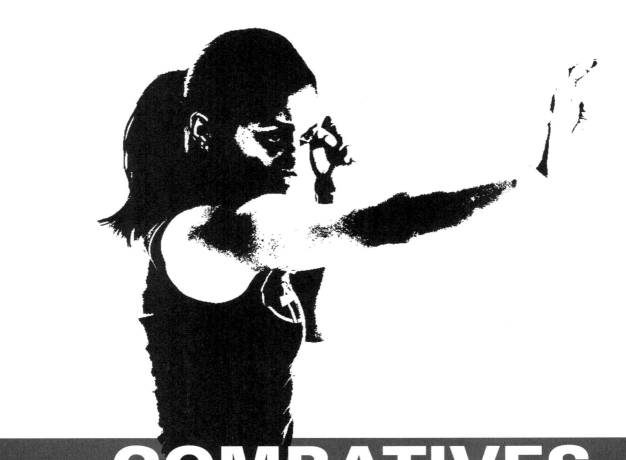

COMBATIVES

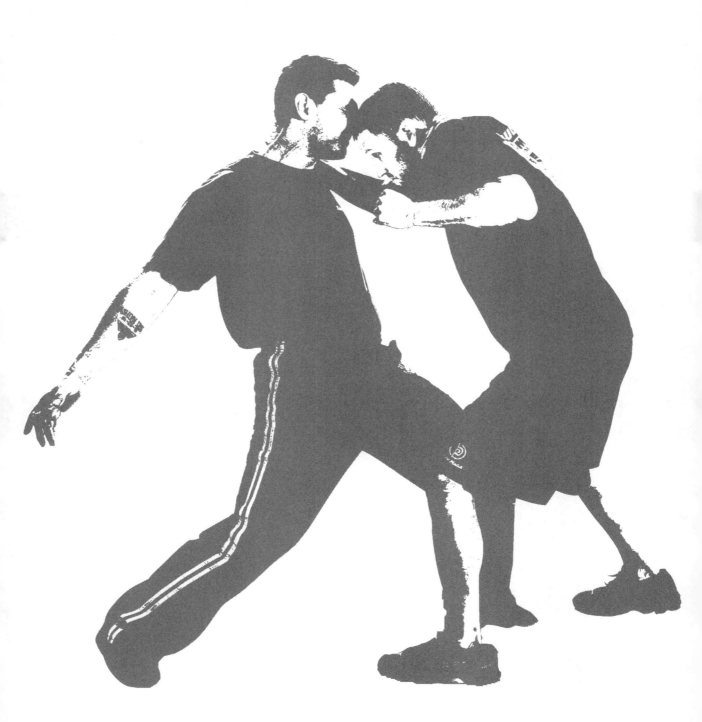

Combatives Overview

Krav Maga refers to techniques that are designed to cause damage and end conflicts as combatives. These techniques are most often categorized as punches, knees, kicks, elbows, headbutts, and the like, although any strike, grab, bite, or other personal weapon is classified as a combative. Combatives are like tools in a tool box. While a few certain tools are more often used, it's best to have others available just in case the need arises.

As stated, the primary goal of combatives is to interrupt the on-going attack. Krav Maga emphasizes the use of multiple combatives in order to overwhelm the assailant. This approach causes a shift in the predator vs. prey mentality, rendering the attacker unwilling or unable to continue the fight, even if just momentarily to facilitate escape. The ability to generate enough power in combatives is made possible through the use and understanding of physics. Proper technique in training allows the transfer of force from the defender to the attacker, turning the defender from "victim to victor."

Combatives are categorized according to ranges. In order to be successful in a fight or self-defense situation, it's important to be versed in all ranges. While some ranges could be broken down into sub-ranges, this book will describe four primary categories.

Long Range. Combatives in this range are typically kicks, which are not only the longest weapon but also the strongest. The opportunity to use combatives in this range often indicates the recognition of a threat early in the conflict or in the finishing or escaping stage of the conflict.

Intermediate Range. This range is normally characterized as "punching range," although this is slightly misleading since other combatives are utilized in this range and some punches are not. Intermediate combatives, such as straight punches, palm heel strikes, hammerfists, and eye strikes, are most effective when the arm is able to reach full extension.

Close Range. Most attacks and threats occur in this range, where an attacker can intimidate, choke, bearhug, headlock, or otherwise grab the defender. Combatives in this range include hook and uppercut punches, elbows, knees, headbutts, and stomps. Other effective combatives in this range may include hair grabs, bites, and gouges, although these weapons are typically more prevalent in groundfighting.

Groundfighting Range. Combatives in this range are essentially the same as those in close range, although the setting, posture, and leverage are different. It's important to note that Krav Maga makes a distinction between groundfighting and grappling, in that the goals of each are different. While groundfighting certainly incorporates techniques from grappling, it's designed to get the defender up and away as soon as possible. Aggressive combatives, coupled with a basic understanding of positions, is the most efficient way to accomplish this goal.

Where to strike

In Krav Maga, students are encouraged to strike vulnerable areas of the attacker's body. This allows smaller defenders to use inherent human weaknesses to render attackers unable or unwilling to continue fighting or, at the very least, facilitate escape.

While there are many vulnerable targets on the body, Krav Maga basic training tends to emphasize the groin, eyes, throat, liver, chin/jaw, and knees. Additional viable targets include kidneys, instep, solar plexus, ears, fingers, and other joints. The diagram below illustrates the location of these preferred targets.

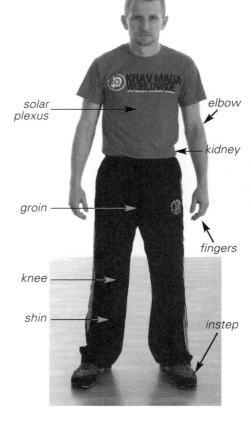

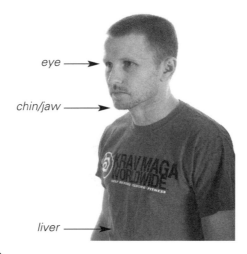

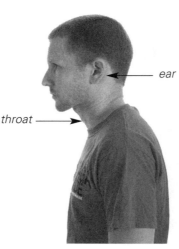

Straight Punch Mechanics

Straight punches may be performed with either the lead hand or the rear hand. Although the word "jab" sometimes creeps into our vocabulary, we try not to use it. A "jab" in boxing is, by design, a weaker punch that is used to score points or set up a stronger cross. On the street you're not fighting for points. We want your forward-hand punch (for most of us, that's the left) to be as strong as possible. To ensure this, make sure your fighting stance is squared up to the opponent. That is, your shoulders and hips are facing almost totally forward. Of course, your left side will be a little bit in front because of your stance and thus your forward punch won't be quite as strong as your rear punch, but you should still work to put as much power into that forward hand as possible.

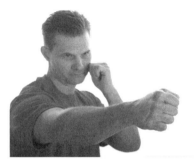
Proper form: wrist is straight.

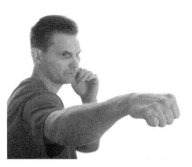
Improper form: wrist is bent.

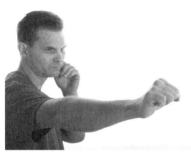
Improper form: wrist is bent outward.

Training Tips

In order to punch with maximum power (especially when throwing a punch from the rear hand), it's important to use your core and legs to drive the motion. Think of it like throwing a ball as far as possible: engage your hips and legs, and then your arm, in order to generate power. Punching effectively is similar. To engage your rear leg, pivot that back foot. It helps to imagine squashing a bug or putting out a cigarette. When punching, it's also important to think in terms of punching through the target, not to it.

In order to cause maximum damage to the attacker and diminish the chances of hand injuries, make impact with the first two knuckles of the fist. Just before impact, rotate the fist to approximately 45 degrees while keeping the wrist straight.

In order to minimize the risk of being punched while punching, tuck your chin to your chest, allowing the shoulder of your punching arm to protect your chin and jaw while keeping your non-punching hand high to your face.

If you notice that your elbow is coming up or out with the punch, stand next to a wall while punching. This method with give you instant feedback and help you to correct this problem. Why keep your elbow down on a straight punch? There are several reasons:

—The punch is harder for your opponent to see.

—The punch travels in a straight line, which is the shortest distance to the target.

—The movement lines up the first two knuckles with the target; lifting your elbow causes the weaker pinky side of your fist to travel toward the target, which may result in a "boxer's fracture."

1-2 Roll your fingers tightly so that there is no space.

3 Seal your thumb tightly over your fingers near the first knuckle. Do NOT put your thumb inside your fingers!

Training Tips: You should never keep a tight fist during an entire fight. You will exhaust yourself and clench your arm muscles, which slows you down. Keep your hands fairly loose until the moment of impact. Then, just before contact, you should make your fist as tight as possible. If there is any air or space inside your first, the fingers will collapse. This robs the punch of some power by absorbing the force, and may lead to possible injury. Make your fist like a rock, not a shock absorber!

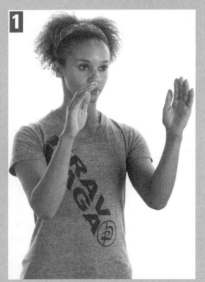

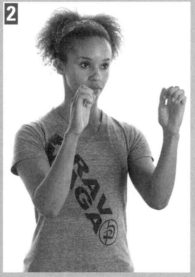

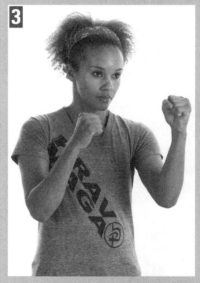

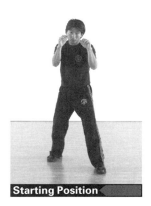

Starting Position

Starting Position: Left-leg-forward fighting stance.

1 Driving with your legs and your core, send your left fist forward.

2 As your hips and shoulders rotate, extend your arm for the punch, keeping your elbow down towards the floor. This increases power and reach.

3 Traveling on the same line, recoil your hand and body quickly back to starting position. This protects your head and prepares you for subsequent punches.

To make a Right Straight Punch, follow the same procedure with your right hand. For most of us, the right hand will be the rear hand and will have more power because the rear hip can pivot forward more powerfully.

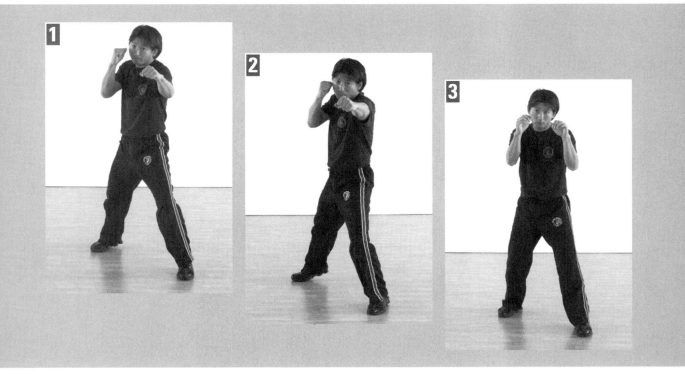

Straight Punch with Advance

You can make any straight punch while advancing to cover distance. Begin practicing with a forward hand, then try other punches while advancing.

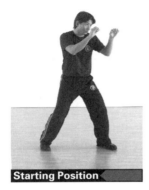

Starting Position

Starting Position: Left-leg-forward fighting stance.

1 Driving with your legs and keeping your elbow down as long as possible, extend your left fist forward. As your hand travels out, rotate your shoulder and hip forward to add power.

2 Immediately burst in with an advance, pushing off with your right foot and moving forward with your left foot. As the punch lands, close the distance by bringing your right foot forward.

Training Tips: Many beginners have trouble with advancing punches because Krav Maga places a lot of emphasis on the weapon being the first thing to move. In other words, we DON'T want you to burst forward and then punch, because you would be making a big body movement (that the opponent can see) without your hand traveling at all. You will speed up your training if you understand that the punch doesn't have to be a movement that is way out in front of the body. It just has to precede the body movement enough so that, by the time your opponent sees your body move, the punch is at least a little closer to the target.

The very best method for learning this technique is with a very small advance. Start with the target just barely out of your reach so that you only need to burst forward a little bit to reach it. Practice the advance at this range until you feel comfortable, then slowly increase the distance. You should never make the distance too great. Remember, at a certain distance, you should be kicking rather than punching…and at an even greater distance, you should probably be looking for a weapon, instead of a punch, to hit him with.

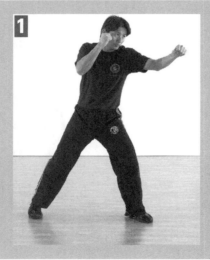

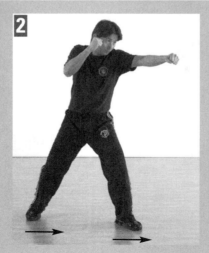

A straight punch can be delivered low—to the midsection or even to the groin.

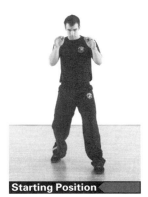

Starting Position

Starting Position: Left-leg-forward fighting stance.

1-2 Extend your right fist forward, sending your fist low while dropping your body by bending at the waist and knees. Do not leave your head up while punching down—this would leave you too exposed. Do not simply drop your body down before sending the punch—this telegraphs the movement. As you drop your head down, move it slightly to the side so that you are not in line with his punches. Be sure to recoil your punch!

Training Tips: Straight punches to the body definitely have their pros and cons. On the one hand, they can be a big surprise for an opponent who is worried mostly about protecting his face and head. On the other, many opponents can absorb a body shot better than they can absorb a punch to the face (unless you hit the solar plexus or liver), so you may not do as much damage. If the fight lasts more than a few seconds, the investment may be worth the risk. Changing heights and targets can confuse the opponent and make him worry about many things at once. The bottom line is this: If you're going to try a low straight punch, be sure you follow the directions here, keep your chin tucked, and take your head off line.

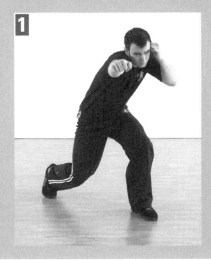

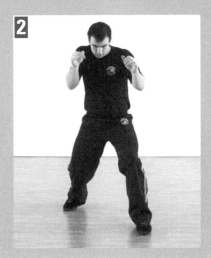

The mechanics of a palm heel strike are the same as a straight punch; all that changes is the striking surface. The comments below apply to either a forward- or rear-hand punch.

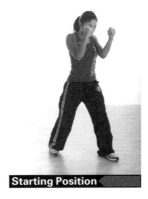

Starting Position ◀

Starting Position: Left-leg-forward fighting stance.

1 Extend your right hand forward, keeping your elbow down as long as possible, and drive with your legs. As your hand travels out, rotate your shoulder and hip forward to add power. Pivot on your back foot.

2 As your hand is about to strike the target, flex your wrist backward, open your hand, and curl your fingers slightly, making contact with the hard surface at the base of your hand. Rotate your wrist inward as you strike—this adds extra power and helps protect your wrist.

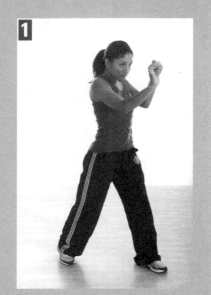

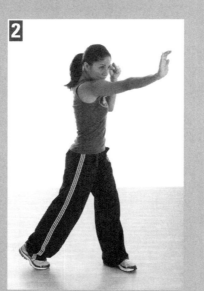

Training Tips: By moving your fingers out of the way, you force the heel of your hand, rather than your fingers, to make contact. If you don't rotate, your wrist may be bent backward on impact, potentially causing a sprain or break.

Elbow Strike Mechanics

Elbows are effective weapons at close range, and can be delivered at almost any angle with power. Keep in mind that there are more than seven elbow strikes. There are, in fact, a nearly infinite number of angles. However, we teach seven elbows as a way of communicating the general movements to beginners. As you train more, you will find variations on these angles based on your position and the position of your opponent.

The striking surface for the elbows is a small surface area just above or below the tip of your bent elbow. Try to strike with the smallest surface possible so that the force of your strike is concentrated. This creates maximum penetration and damage. Also, for all elbow strikes, bring your hand to your shoulder, creating a sharp bend in the elbow itself. Your hand can be closed in a fist or slightly curled at the fingers—whatever is most comfortable for you. Be aware that if you close your fist too tightly, you will tighten up the muscles of your arm and reduce your speed.

For training purposes, we show elbows only with the right hand, but of course the left elbow can be delivered from all the same angles. Also, for all of these elbows, you should begin with what we'll call a "modified neutral stance." That is, a neutral stance, but with your hands up. This facilitates the training. Later, you can step into a fighting stance and train from there as well.

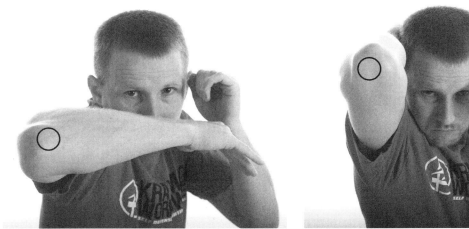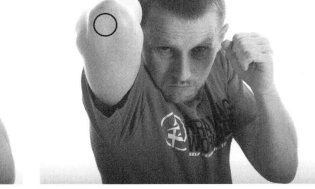

The striking surface for both of these elbow strikes is just above the tip of the elbow.

Horizontal High Elbow Strike (Elbow #1)

This elbow strike targets an attacker coming from the front.

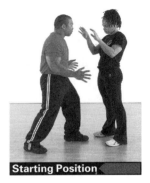

Starting Position

Starting Position: Modified neutral stance with both hands up.

1 Bring your right hand in to your shoulder, creating a firm bend in your elbow.

2 Sharply swing your elbow out horizontally in front of you to make contact with your target's face or throat. Strike with the point just below the tip of your elbow, pivoting as you strike to generate more power.

Recoil and return to starting position.

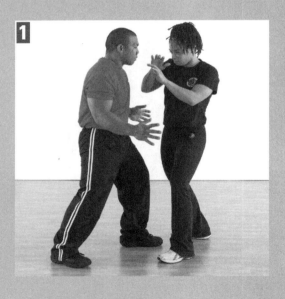

1

Training Tips: Beginners are sometimes confused by the angle of this attack. This elbow can be delivered in a circular motion (traveling in front of your body from right to left) or in a forward motion (traveling outward like a straight punch), depending on the position of the target.

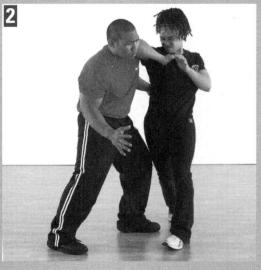

2

Sideways Elbow Strike (Elbow #2)

This elbow strike targets an attacker coming from the side.

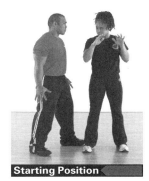

Starting Position

Starting Position: Modified neutral stance with both hands up.

1 Bring your right hand in to your shoulder, creating a firm bend in your elbow. Raise your elbow up.

2 Strike to the side, avoiding a "flapping" motion. Lean in as you strike, making contact just above the tip of your elbow. Use your legs for power.

Recoil and return to starting position.

Training Tips: The most common mistake beginners make is forgetting to add power by using their legs and body. Be careful not to simply "poke" with your elbow itself—drive through with your legs.

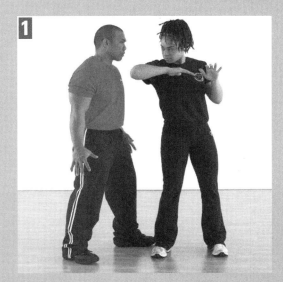

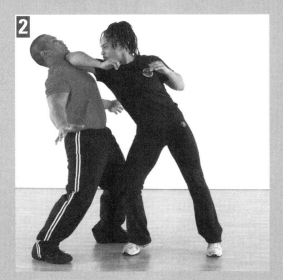

This elbow strike targets an attacker coming from behind.

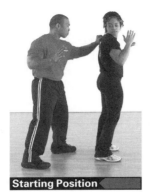

Starting Position

Starting Position: Modified neutral stance with both hands up.

1 Bring your right hand in to your shoulder, creating a firm bend in your elbow.

2 Pivot as you punch your elbow horizontally to a target behind you, looking back over your shoulder to see your target; make sure to keep your chin tucked for protection. Strike with the point just above the tip of your elbow.

Recoil and return to starting position.

Training Tips: This is a very powerful elbow that you will use often when learning bearhug defenses. Make it a comfortable part of your arsenal.

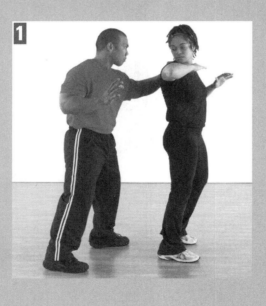

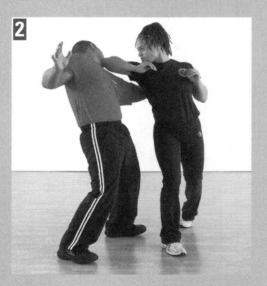

Vertical Elbow Strike Backward Low (Elbow #4)

This elbow strike targets an attacker coming from behind.

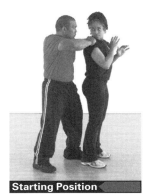

Starting Position

Starting Position: Modified neutral stance with both hands up.

1 Send your elbow straight back to make contact with your target's ribs or stomach. Strike with the point just above the tip of your elbow, pivoting as you strike to generate more power.

Recoil and return to starting position.

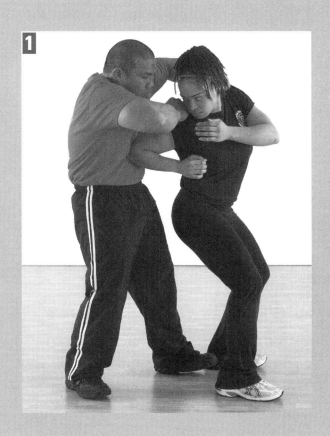

Training Tips: It's good to practice this elbow by keeping your arm close to your body. Assume that someone is trying to grab you in a bearhug from behind. If you swing your arm away from your body as you strike backward, you may find your arm blocked. Think of your forearm brushing along your ribs.

Vertical Elbow Strike Backward (Elbow #5)

This elbow strike targets an attacker coming from behind.

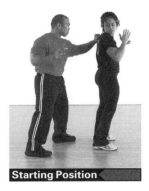

Starting Position

Starting Position: Modified neutral stance with both hands up.

1 Bring your right hand in to your shoulder, creating a firm bend in your elbow.

2-3 Punch your elbow backward and upward, tilting your shoulders forward to strike the attacker's throat or face. Strike with the point just above the tip of your elbow.

Recoil and return to starting position.

Training Tips: This elbow is very similar to #4—just tilt forward slightly so that your elbow drives upward instead of straight back. In a real fight, the act of tilting forward also creates a little space between you and your attacker, giving your elbow room to drive upward forcefully.

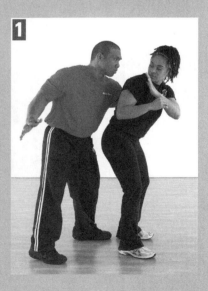

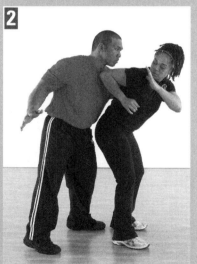

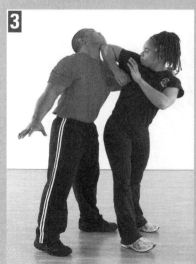

Vertical Elbow Strike Forward and Upward (Elbow #6)

This elbow strike targets an attacker coming from the front.

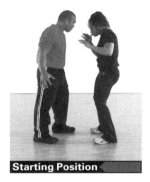

Starting Position

Starting Position: Modified neutral stance with both hands up.

1 Bring your right hand in to your shoulder, creating a firm bend in your elbow.

2-3 Swing your elbow up, pivoting your hip and shoulder in and up to generate more power. Strike your target's chin with the point just below the tip of your elbow.

Recoil and return to starting position.

Training Tips: A great analogy for this movement is to think of brushing your hair back from your ear. This helps you to drive your elbow straight upward. Some students have limited range of motion and may not be able to rotate their arm and shoulder upward fully. You can vary this movement by raising your arm diagonally across your body so that your elbow travels up and across to the other side. This variation may not help you strike at all openings, but it's better than not striking at all.

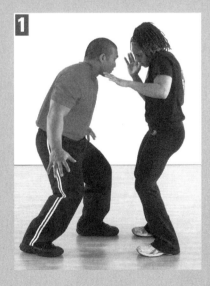

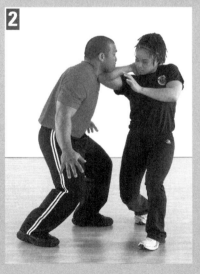

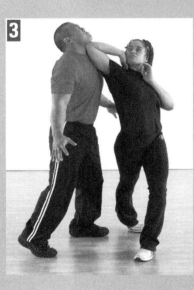

Vertical Elbow Strike Forward and Down (Elbow #7)

This elbow strike is similar to a downward hammerfist (page 91). The attacker is poised to attack you from a low angle, or is doubled over (following a groin kick, for example).

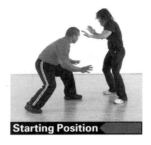

Starting Position

Starting Position: Modified neutral stance with both hands up.

1 Bring your right hand in to your shoulder, creating a firm bend in your elbow.

2 Bend your knees and drop your weight down as you swing your elbow down. Strike the back of your opponent's head or neck with the point just above (i.e., toward your shoulder) the tip of your elbow.

Recoil and return to starting position.

Training Tips: If you're going to use this elbow in a real violent encounter, be sure you target sensitive areas. Don't try giving this elbow to your opponent's back. He won't feel it during an adrenaline rush. Target areas that will hurt him immediately so that you can be safe.

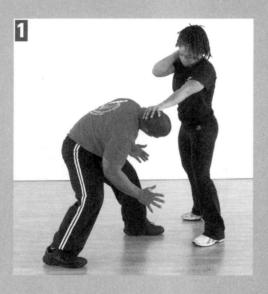

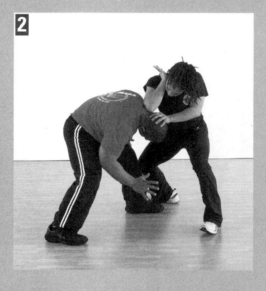

A hook punch is suitable when your opponent is close. Rather than punching straight ahead, you bend your elbow and punch around your opponent's defense, aiming at the side of his face or body. Body movement is extremely important. Here we demonstrate a left hook punch, but you can execute a right hook punch as well. In some ways, a right hook punch is easier because it's easier to engage the rear hip.

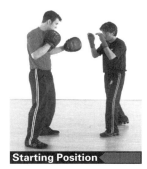

Starting Position

Starting Position: Left-leg-forward fighting stance.

1 Send your left fist forward, bringing your elbow up so that your forearm is parallel to the floor. Your elbow should remain bent. As your hand travels to the target, the meaty part (the pinky end of the fist) should remain down. Rotate your left shoulder and hip forward and inward, adding power in the direction of the punch. Make contact with your first two knuckles against the side of your opponent's jaw or body. Pivot the front (left) foot to add power.

2 Recoil. The fastest way to recover from the hook punch is to simply drop your elbow down (this brings your hand up into a guard position) then rotate your body back into starting position.

Training Tips: A hook punch is very similar to Elbow #1. As you train more, you'll notice that you can deliver hook punches from many angles and distances. When your opponent is very close, throw a hook punch with a very bent elbow. When he is farther away, open your elbow up so the hook punch reaches farther in front of you.

Be sure your elbow and forearm are supporting your fist. If your punch is traveling exactly parallel to the floor, then your forearm should be exactly parallel to the floor. This allows your forearm to brace your hand when your fist strikes the target, adding power and protecting your hand.

One trick to learning a good hook punch is to relax your shoulder as much as possible. Some beginners make their shoulder very rigid so that the arm moves only in association with the body rotation. Relax your shoulder so that the arm can move independently of the body. Then, when the body turns and the arm swings, the two motions act to create even more power.

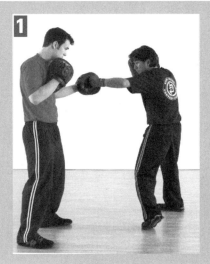

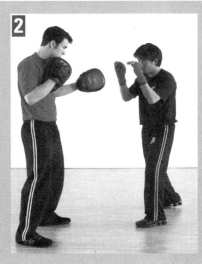

An uppercut can be thought of as a hook punch from a different angle. Whereas the body rotates inward in the direction of the hook punch, the uppercut punch rotates the body upward.

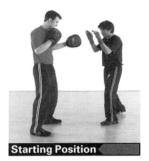

Starting Position

Starting Position: Left-leg-forward fighting stance.

1 Bend slightly at the waist (contracting your abs) and knees. This will drop your center a bit below the target. The amount of bend can be very slight, depending on the height of your opponent—your only goal is to get your punching hand below the target without lowering your hands too far from your face.

2 Punch out and upward with your left hand so that the meaty part of your fist faces your opponent's body. Rotate your left shoulder inward and upward. Keep your elbow close to your body at all times. Do not drop your hand down to your waist—this exposes you to a counter punch. As your punch rises toward the target, drive your legs upward as well, adding power. Just before contact, rotate your fist so that your palm faces back toward you, adding torque to the punch.

Once you've punched through the target, pull your arm back down in a piston-like motion to recoil and return to starting position.

Training Tips: When you make an uppercut punch, think about your elbow sliding along your ribs. This encourages you to strike straight upward, rather than on an awkward diagonal, which is a common mistake. If you rip straight up the middle, your punch will be stronger and harder for the opponent to see.

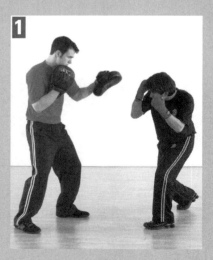

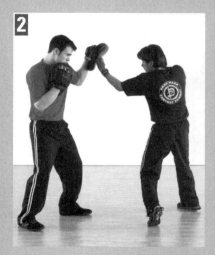

Forward Headbutt

A headbutt can be a devastating weapon; it's performed at extremely close range, either while standing or on the ground. Be sure to keep your chin down and strike with the crown of your forehead against the soft tissue of his face. In this book, we only cover the headbutt forward. There are more angles at which you can use a headbutt, but this is by far the most common.

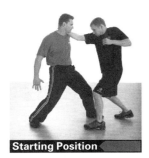

Starting Position

Starting Position: Stand nearly toe to toe with your opponent. You can grab your opponent's head, either by the ears or sides of the hair, for extra control and power.

1 Keeping your neck stiff and your jaw tightly closed, drive your head forward using your legs and upper body. The striking surface is the top of your forehead, right at the hair line. The target should be the attacker's nose, cheekbone, etc.

Training Tips: It's not necessary to grab the face or head. A powerful (and sneaky) headbutt can be delivered without the grab. If you do grab, be careful not to pull the attacker's chin downward. This hides his face and exposes the hard skull, which will damage you. We have seen people knock themselves out giving headbutts this way.

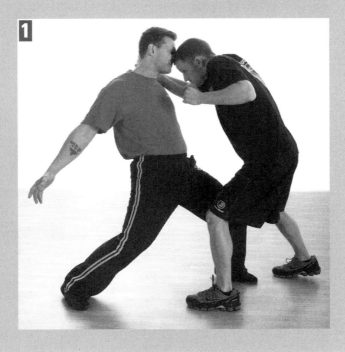

Hammerfist Punch

Just like elbows, hammerfist punches can be delivered at almost any angle with power. When training hammerfist punches, you may want to use a neutral stance so that you can focus on turning your hips for power. The striking surface for all hammerfist punches is the pinky side of the fist, also called the "meat" part of the fist. While a regular punch runs some risk of injury to the knuckles, the hammerfist strike is very safe. Hammerfist punches are most effective to the face or back of the neck.

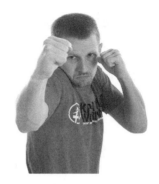

Hammerfist to the Side

Hammerfist to the side may be practiced from a fighting stance or a neutral stance. Because it's often used in reaction to a surprise attack, we generally present the strike from a passive stance first.

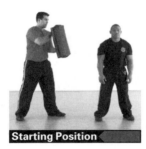

Starting Position

Starting Position: Passive stance.

1 Move your right hand sideways and upward, elbow slightly bent. As your hand moves toward its target, rotate your hip and shoulder. Tuck your chin. Your rising arm should cover you as well as strike. Pivot your outside foot and step in toward your target to make sure weight is being transferred into the punch.

2 On contact, your elbow should still be somewhat bent. The bent elbow should pass your target to help the punch penetrate; it also helps prevent hyperextension of the joint.

Recoil and return to starting position.

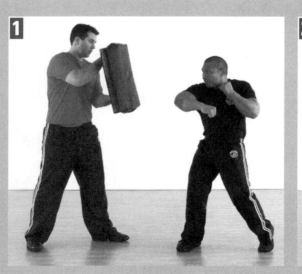

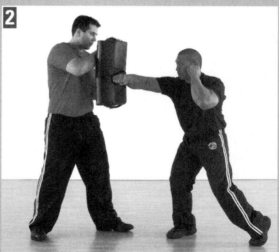

Hammerfist to the Back

Hammerfist to the back is essentially the same as hammerfist to the side, but with a greater turn to meet an attack coming from behind. You should practice it to develop the concept that you can strike in a full circle around your body.

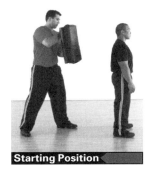

Starting Position

Starting Position: Passive stance.

1 Look over your right shoulder, but keep your chin tucked. Move your right hand sideways and upward, elbow slightly bent. As your hand moves toward its target, rotate your hip and shoulder. Your rising arm should cover you as well as strike. Pivot your outside foot and step in toward your target to make sure weight is being transferred into the punch.

2 On contact, your elbow should still be somewhat bent. The bent elbow should pass your target to help the punch penetrate; it also helps prevent hyperextension of the joint.

Recoil and return to starting position.

Training Tips: Make sure the movement on hammerfist to the back covers your face. It's not a defensive movement—it's an attack!—but it should offer you some coverage in case the opponent's attack reaches you first.

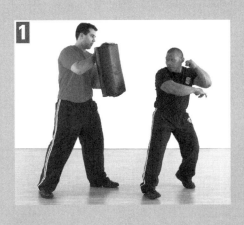

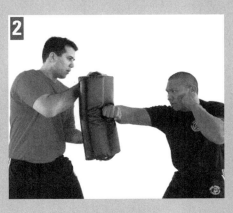

A forward hammerfist is generally a strike to your opponent's face.

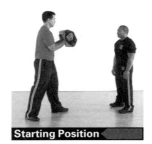

Starting Position

Starting Position: Passive stance.

1 Raise your right hand in a small windup—roughly from chin height to about eyebrow height. Don't throw your hand too high above your head—that motion would be too slow and detectable.

2 As your fist comes down, generate power by rotating your shoulder and hip inward and forward while driving with your legs.

Recoil and return to starting position.

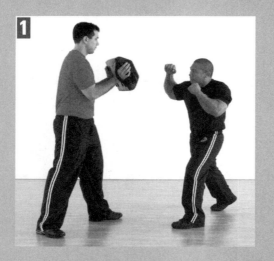

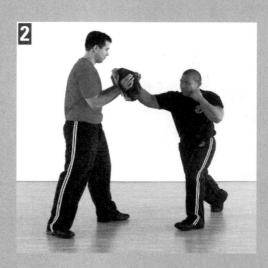

Downward Hammerfist

A downward hammerfist will generally be to the back of your opponent's neck, at the base of the skull with your opponent doubled over (for example, after a groin kick). Other targets may be the kidneys (against a low bearhug) or face.

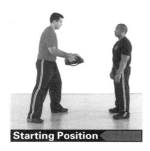

Starting Position

Starting Position: Passive stance.

1 Raise your right fist upward in a small windup.

2 As your punch descends, generate power by rotating your hip and shoulder inward and down, and by bending your knees. Do not bend at the waist.

Recoil and return to starting position.

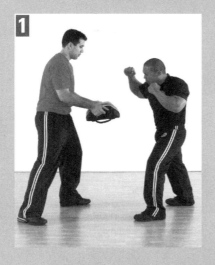

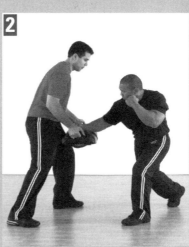

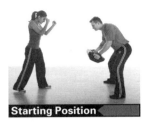

Starting Position

Fighting Stance

Starting Position: Left-leg-forward fighting stance.

1 Swing your right leg forward, bending your knee.

2 As your hip comes forward and upward, snap your foot out, driving through the target. Pivot slightly on your left (base) foot—this opens your hips, which helps extend the kick and add power. The striking surface can either be your instep, about where you tie your shoelaces, or your shin.

Recoil. After making contact, you should be able to either put the kicking foot down in front of you or bring it back into a fighting stance.

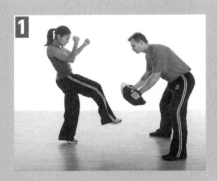

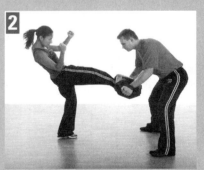

Training Tips: The comment about pivoting slightly with your base foot is very important, especially if you aren't very flexible. To gain power in the kick, your hips must open forward. For those of us who are less flexible, the slight pivot of the base foot will give your hips room to open. Also, as stated, you can strike with either the instep or the shin. The shin is much stronger, but the instep can be useful when the target is a little farther away.

If you were to kick from a neutral stance, there is no real difference as far as the kicking leg is concerned. However, because your body is not ready to deliver a kick, you may add the following training tip: To gain power from a neutral stance, shift your weight suddenly and explosively to the base foot and send your kicking leg sharply toward the target. If you make the motion too slow (i.e., "shift 1, kick 2"), you will telegraph the kick. The weight shift and kick should happen simultaneously. Also, emphasize speed and penetration over power. Although we always want to deliver a strong strike, even a lighter groin kick can do damage as long as it hits the target!

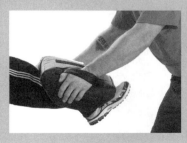

Front Kick (Vertical Target)

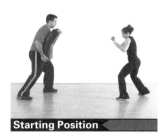

Starting Position

Starting Position: Left-leg-forward fighting stance.

1 Bring your right leg forward and your knee up.

2 Punch the foot, leg, and hip straight out (i.e., not upward, as in the front kick to the groin). As you kick, curl your toes upward to the top of your shoe, exposing and tightening the ball of your foot. Strike with the ball of your foot.

Recoil. You should be able to make a strong kick and then plant your kicking foot to any point, as needed, either in front or recovering back to a fighting stance.

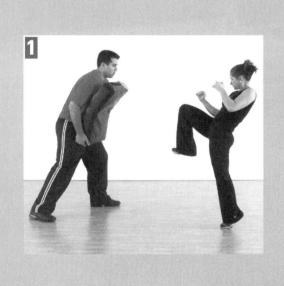

Training Tips: Although this kick does rise from the ground (since your feet start on the ground), the general motion is horizontal so that you can strike a vertical target such as the opponent's stomach.

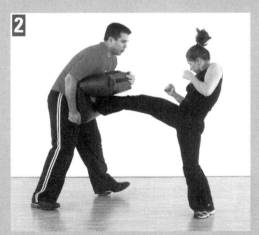

A round kick is, essentially, a front kick that "rolls over" at the last minute. Like the regular front kick, the round kick uses your instep or shin as the striking surface. In a more advanced version, you make contact with the ball of your foot. Round kick can be made to the side of an opponent's knee joint, thigh, ribs, or even head, although we do not emphasize high kicks in Krav Maga.

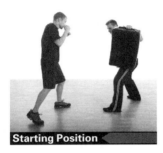

Starting Position

Starting Position: Left-leg-forward fighting stance.

1 Raise your right knee almost exactly as you would for a front kick. However, as the kick rises, roll your hips inward so that the kick changes to a horizontal motion. It will help to pivot on the ball of your base foot so that the heel of your base foot turns forward.

2-3 As your hips pivot, "chop" your leg onto the target and continue rolling your hip. Be sure to penetrate. Your knee should retain some bend even on contact to protect against hyperextension.

Recoil. You should be able to land forward with control, or bring your foot back into a fighting stance.

Training Tips: When you send this kick, be sure you are in a good position to swing your leg through the target, rather than just touching the outer surface of the target. For instance, if you're kicking with your right leg, your body should be centered on the target so that you break through it. If you're too far to the right, your kick will have lost its power by the time it arrives on target. If you start a little more to the left, your kick will penetrate more deeply and do more damage.

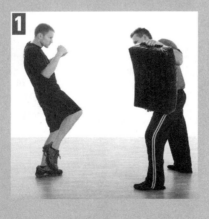

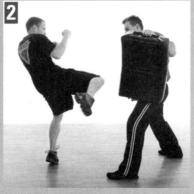

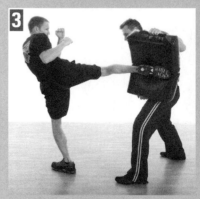

Think of a back kick as a stomp. You make contact with the bottom of your heel. Practice back kick first while in place, then practice it with a small step.

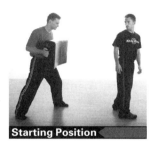

Starting Position

Starting Position: Passive stance. The target is behind you. First, recognize the threat with a brief, natural glance over your shoulder.

1-2 Chamber your right knee in front of you, then send your right foot backward, toes down (not pointed), toward the target. Make contact with your heel going into the target. At the same time, bend your body forward and shift your hips (especially the kicking side) backward into the kick. As you kick, look around your arm, not over your shoulder. If you continue looking over your shoulder, you'll be unable to bend and shift your weight into the kick.

Recoil. As a beginner, you may end up with your back to the target. Once you've mastered the kick, recoil while pivoting on your left (base) foot so that you're facing the target.

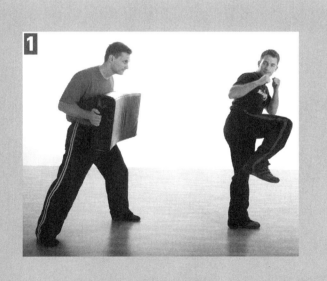

Training Tips: One of the simplest ways to introduce the mechanics of a back kick is to imagine stomping an aluminum can. Raise your knee up in front of your body and stomp down on the imaginary can, using your heel. You will naturally put some weight behind the stomp by driving your hip down into the motion. Now, keep that motion in mind and make the same stomp…only this time backwards.

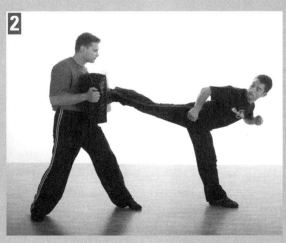

Unlike Front Kick to a Vertical Target (page 93), which is designed to penetrate and cause damage, the main purpose of a defensive front kick is to either stop an advancing opponent or to push a close opponent to a greater distance. For this reason, we kick with the whole foot. More surface area means the kick will push more than penetrate.

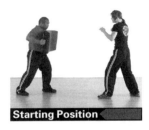

Starting Position

Starting Position: Left-leg-forward fighting stance.

1 Bring your right knee up high, with your toes flexed back (not pointed). Send your foot forward, stomping with the entire foot. On contact, your knee should still be slightly bent to protect against hyperextension. Be sure to drive your right hip into the kick, and also engage your base leg for more power.

Recoil (either forward or back) quickly.

Training Tips: Although Krav Maga tries to reduce the importance of timing in its techniques, there is some timing involved here. If you kick too early, you may hyperextend your knee. If you kick too late against an approaching opponent, you may jam your kick and get knocked backward. Always practice the kick against a stationery target first, and then against a slowly advancing target, so that you learn to gauge your distance.

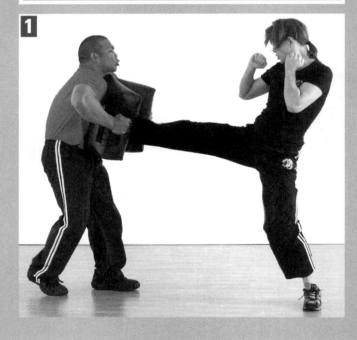

Knee strikes are to kicks as elbows are to straight punches. That is, they are essentially the same strike done at a shorter distance.

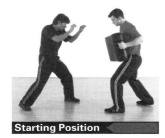

Starting Position

Starting Position: Left-leg-forward fighting stance in close proximity to your opponent.

1 With your left hand, grab your opponent's right arm somewhere around the elbow or upper arm. With your right hand, catch his shoulder and neck firmly by grabbing handfuls of skin. Push your right forearm against your opponent's neck, keeping your elbow down. This prevents your opponent from dropping down and "shooting in" to grab your legs.

2 Pull your opponent's body forward and/or down while bringing your right knee up sharply, striking the groin, midsection, or face with the point just above your kneecap. Drive your hip forward and up to generate power.

Training Tips: One common mistake that beginners make is to throw their whole body at the opponent. This feels aggressive because they feel themselves burst toward the opponent. However, there is very little power in the knee itself. Instead, drive your knee and hip forward and into the attacker. This is much stronger, and also allows you to retain better balance and control your distance in the fight.

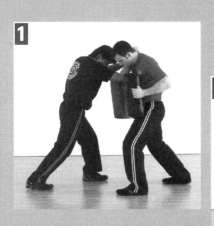

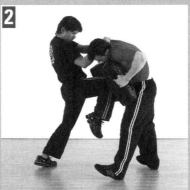

Knee strikes may be applied from different angles. Like a round kick, a round knee starts like the standard strike—relatively straight, and then the hip rolls over. This variation should be practiced after you've mastered the basic knee strike; it's quite effective if your opponent is in front of you but leaves his side open to your attack.

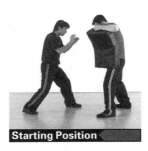

Starting Position

Starting Position: Left-leg-forward fighting stance in close proximity to your opponent.

1 Grab your opponent's right arm and shoulder firmly by grabbing handfuls of skin. Push your right forearm against your opponent's neck, keeping your elbow down. This prevents your opponent from dropping down and "shooting in" to grab your legs.

2 Pull your opponent's body forward and/or down while bringing your right knee up; roll your hip over in a motion similar to a round kick so that your knee strikes at a more horizontal angle. This strike is normally delivered to the ribs, stomach, or head. Drive your hip forward and up to generate power.

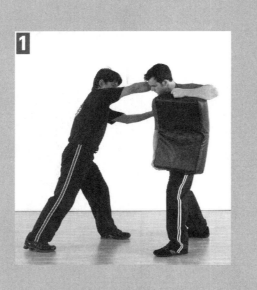

1

Training Tips: As you learn to deliver both knees, do some slow training exercises with a partner (or a heavy bag) in which you stand close and learn to give both forward knees and round knees, making light contact but always emphasizing the extension of your hip into the strike.

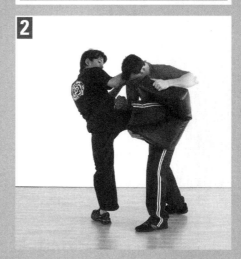

2

DEFENSES

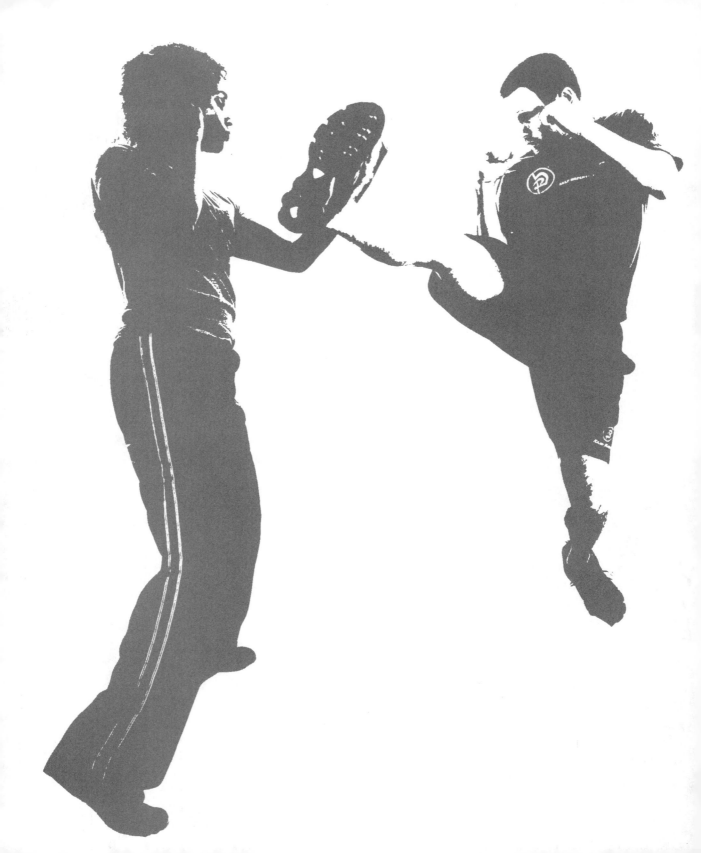

Defenses Overview

The self-defense sections are organized by types of by attack. Each attack is then broken down by *immediate danger, secondary dangers, solution, initial counterattack, neutralizing the attacker, key points,* and *commonly asked questions*. Many defenses will also be accompanied by supplementary teaching tips to further explain the techniques.

Attack is relatively self-explanatory. This is the action taken by the assailant. Defenders should train in a position of disadvantage, often referred to as "neutral," as previously discussed. The **immediate danger** refers to the real problem of the attack, and what the nature of the attack is designed to do. **Secondary dangers** are problems that may arise as a follow-up to the primary danger or as a result of the initial defense.

The **solution** is the defense itself. This is the technique or response that addresses the immediate danger, while the **initial counterattack** is the combative designed to stop the ongoing attack. The initial counterattack is what shifts the dynamics of the fight, and it should be delivered simultaneously to the solution or defense, if possible.

Neutralizing the attacker refers to combatives that follow the initial defense and counter in order to render the attacker unable or unwilling to continue fighting and facilitate escape. Krav Maga recognizes that follow-up combatives should be based on the reaction of the attacker, as opposed to some predetermined sequence of strikes or events. Again, Krav Maga is about problem solving. For example, training to throw a groin kick and then a headbutt is likely not going to be effective or advised in most instances because of the natural reaction to the groin kick. Slow fighting, where a student performs counterattacks at a greatly reduced speed, is often a valuable tool here. It helps students to learn tool and target acquisition (in other words, which vital areas are exposed, and which combatives are most efficient in the moment). Remember, even in slow fighting, the initial pluck should *always* be performed explosively.

In order to provide a quick reference and review, **key points** are provided at the end of each section, along with **commonly asked questions**. This section is another key aspect of Krav Maga that differentiates it from other styles or systems. Krav Maga not only welcomes but encourages students to ask questions. This philosophy is how Krav Maga has improved over the years, and how it will continue to improve in years to come. Krav Maga instructors are concerned with preserving lives, not ego or tradition.

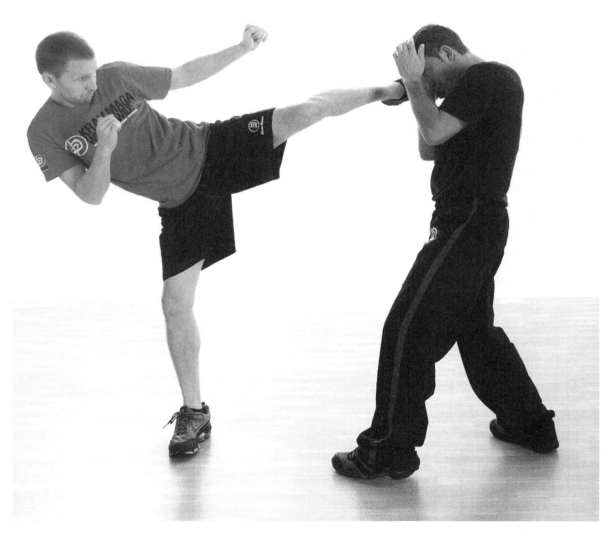

This exercise serves as a basic introduction to outside defenses. "Outside defenses" refer to any defense where our arms move outward, away from the center of our body, and are usually performed against attacks coming from the outside inward, such as hook punches, round kicks, and, later, knife defenses. While the wide attacks used to practice 360 are not the most practical, they do occur on the street. In addition, these attacks are an excellent way for beginners to learn to use not only the defenses, but to develop good vision and fighting spirit. The 360° defenses are based on the body's instinctive reactions and performed with the fingers extended. This is a relatively instinctive (reflexive) movement, which makes it quick; extending your fingers adds a few inches to the defense.

ATTACK The attacker swings his arm downward to the head or collar bone; upward to the groin; or horizontally at the body or head. For training purposes, during these early stages, the attacking arm should be fairly wide and easy to see. The defender should train from a neutral position, but may have his hands up. The attacker may strike lightly, but must put some weight behind each attack in order to test the defense. In addition, every attack should actually strike the defender (lightly) if it's not defended.

With all of the defenses described below, keep the following four principles in mind:
- Keep a 90° bend in your elbow.
- Defend wrist to wrist.
- Use the blade of your arm to defend.
- Defend aggressively, putting weight into your defense (think of attacking the attack).

IMMEDIATE DANGER *Being struck.* The primary danger is being hit.

SECONDARY DANGERS *Disorientation, balance.* If the initial attack is not blocked, the defender may find himself disoriented by the first strike, or knocked off balance, and therefore open to additional strikes.

SOLUTION *360° Defense.* With all these defense positions, make the movement quickly and then recoil.

Starting Position: Neutral stance, hands up at shoulder/face level.

Position 1: With your elbow bent 90°, raise your forearm above and slightly in front of your head to defend against an attack coming straight down.

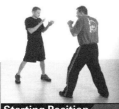

Starting Position

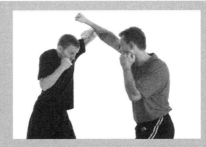

Position 1

continued on next page

continued from previous page

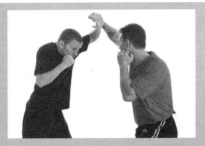

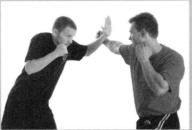

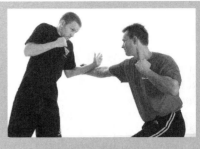

Position 2   *Position 3*   *Position 4*

Position 2: With your elbow bent 90°, raise your arm at an angle (like the roof of a house—about 30°) to defend against an attack at 45°.

Position 3: Starting with your elbow bent 90°, send your forearm out parallel with the floor (with both arms it would look like horizontal goalposts) to defend against an attack coming directly from the side.

Position 4: Bring your elbow (bent 90°) in tight to your body to defend against an upward attack to your ribs. Angle your forearm slightly outward and contract your abs.

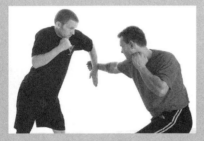

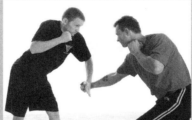

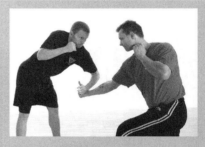

Position 5   *Position 6*   *Position 7*

Position 5: With your elbow bent 90°, point your fingers down to defend against an upward attack to your ribs. This is the exact opposite of Position #3.

Position 6: Starting with your elbow bent 90°, lower your arm at a 30° angle to defend against a rising attack to your body. Be sure to bend at your waist, not at your knees.

Position 7: Starting with your elbow bent 90°, lower your forearm below and slightly in front of your chest to defend against a rising attack to the center of your body. Be sure to bend at your waist, not at your knees.

INITIAL COUNTERATTACK *Straight Punch (page 71).* During your initial training, practice the defenses only. Once you've learned the basic 360° defenses, you can add a simultaneous straight punch. The punch is generally made to the attacker's face.

NEUTRALIZING THE ATTACKER After the initial counterstrike, the defender should continue to strike with elbows to the body and face. Students must focus on rendering the attacker unwilling or unable to continue the assault.

KEY POINTS

- 90° bend in the elbow
- wrist to wrist
- defend using the blade of your arm
- put weight into your defense ("attack the attack")

COMMONLY ASKED QUESTIONS

Why should I keep my fingers extended?
Technically, this makes your defense longer, which gives you a better chance to defend even if you're a little off. More importantly, the 360° defense is reflexive, and reflexive motions are made with open hands or slightly curled fingers, not a real fist. Finally, the more you make a fist, the tighter your forearm muscles will be, which slows down your defense.

Why should I defend "wrist to wrist"?
At this level, defending wrist to wrist gives you the best chance of stopping the attack—if the attack comes lower than you expected, you have your whole forearm available to help block the strike. This is also the foundation of our knife defenses, and, in those defenses, the "wrist to wrist" action helps to control the attacker's knife hand.

Why is it so important to use the blade of the forearm?
It's harder, and hurts the attacker.

Why should I bend at the waist when I make the lower defenses?
Bending at the waist allows you to go down to meet the attack with your arm without bringing your body closer to the attack. If you bend at the knees, your body will come closer to the attack.

What is the difference between #4 and #5? They seem to cover the same area.
These two positions do cover the same area (the lower ribs). Position #4 is generally used when your hands are already up, so all you must do is drop your elbow down a little and contract your abs. Position #5 is often made when your hands are already down, so you only need to raise your elbow.

Training Tips: It's important to realize that the seven positions are only teaching tools. There are, of course, an infinite number of positions and angles between each of the seven we have shown. Remember the key points listed above and you'll be able to defend from any angle of attack.

You should *not* think of these defenses as circular, arcing motions of the forearm, using the elbow as a hinge. (To use a pop culture reference from the movie *Karate Kid*, these are not "wax on, wax off" movements.) Send your entire forearm as one unit, extending from the upper arm and shoulder, rather than "hinging" at the elbow.

ATTACK The attacker throws a right straight punch to the defender's face or throat.

IMMEDIATE DANGER *Being struck.* The primary danger is being hit.

SECONDARY DANGERS *Disorientation, balance.* If the initial attack is not blocked, the defender may find himself disoriented by the first strike, or knocked off balance, and therefore open to additional strikes.

SOLUTION *Inside Defense*

1 As the attack travels forward, use your left hand to redirect the punch (if he punches with his left, you defend with your right). Push your hand, palm open, forward and inward about 45°, but *only* a small distance. Let the punch slide along your palm. This will redirect it slightly away from your face. At the same time, make a small body defense by moving your head to the outside. Be sure to keep your elbow down as you defend. This allows you to defend anywhere from the tip of your elbow up to your fingers, just in case the punch travels higher or lower than you expected.

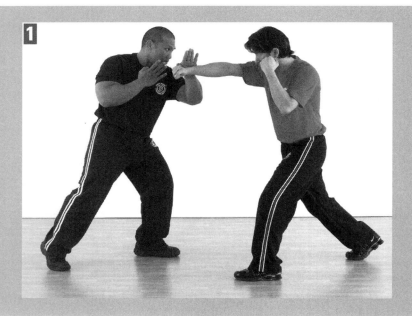

INITIAL COUNTERATTACK *Straight Punch.* During your initial training, practice the defenses only. Once you've learned the basic 360° defenses, you can add a simultaneous straight punch with the other hand. The punch is generally made to the attacker's face.

NEUTRALIZING THE ATTACKER After the initial counterstrike, the defender should continue to strike with elbows to the body and face. Students must focus on rendering the attacker unwilling or unable to continue the assault.

- redirect the punch by letting it slide along your palm
- do not make the motion too big
- make sure your hand travels forward as well as inward
- make a body defense by moving your head slightly to the outside

COMMONLY ASKED QUESTIONS

I keep slapping at the attacker's hand. Is that OK?
No. Slapping usually means you're making too big a motion. Just think of building a ramp and letting the attack slide along your palm or wrist so that it's redirected away.

Do I have to defend with my palm?
The palm is preferred, but it's possible that the punch travels higher or lower than you expected (for instance, you may think he's punching at your nose, but he's really punching at your throat). In that case, you may end up redirecting the punch with your wrist or forearm. This is exactly why we want your elbow to stay down—so that you can defend anywhere along your forearm.

Why not make a bigger defense? Isn't it safer to move the punch farther away?
You only need the punch to miss your face. You don't get bonus points if the punch misses you by a foot rather than an inch. In fact, the farther you move the attacker's punch, the more out of position *your* hand is, which means you must recover from your defense at the same time that he is recovering from his punch. If he's faster, you might lose that race. Making a small defense means that you keep your hands as close to a basic fighting stance is possible, so that you're prepared to deal with any additional attacks that follow that straight punch.

Why is it so important to defend inward and forward? Why not just move the defense laterally across my face?
By moving your hand diagonally forward and inward, you can go out to meet the punch earlier in time and therefore farther from your face. If you move your hand laterally only, then you can only defend the punch as it arrives closer to you.

Training Tips: Practice slowly at first. Have a partner punch you slowly, but with a real punch that would touch you if you did not defend. Prove to yourself how small a defense you can make and still redirect the punch. Feel the punch slide along your palm. Once you feel comfortable with your ability to redirect the punch, have your partner increase the speed of the attack.

Have your partner punch you from a short distance away with a Straight Punch with Advance (page 74). If the attacker is too close to you, you may not have enough time to defend. In any case, in a real fight, if the attacker is that close, you should probably be attacking rather than trying to defend.

Inside Defense against Straight Punch Low

ATTACK The attacker throws a right straight punch to the defender's midsection.

IMMEDIATE DANGER *Being struck.* The primary danger is being hit.

SECONDARY DANGERS *Disorientation, balance.* If the initial attack is not blocked, the defender may find himself disoriented by the first strike, or have the wind knocked out of him, or be knocked off balance, and therefore open to additional strikes.

SOLUTION *Inside Defense (using the forearm or elbow)*

1 As the attack travels forward and down toward the body, use your left hand to redirect the punch (if he punches with his left, you defend with your right); keep your hand up so that you're able to defend your face if the punch comes higher than expected. Lead with your elbow, but bring your entire forearm forward and cross your body, allowing the punch to slide along your forearm. You can get your forearm forward by extending from the shoulder and upper arm. At the same time, make a body defense by turning the defending shoulder and side forward to "blade" your body.

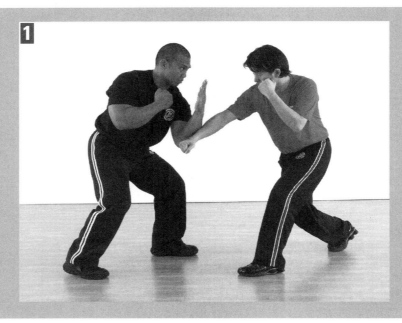

INITIAL COUNTERATTACK *Straight Punch (page 71).* During your initial training, practice the defenses only. Once you've learned the basic inside defenses, you can add a simultaneous straight punch with the other hand. The punch is generally made to the attacker's face.

NEUTRALIZING THE ATTACKER After the initial counterstrike, the defender should continue to strike with elbows to the body and face. Students must focus on rendering the attacker unwilling or unable to continue the assault.

- redirect the punch by letting it slide along your forearm
- do not make the motion too big
- make sure your elbow travels forward as well as inward
- make a body defense by blading your body

COMMONLY ASKED QUESTIONS

I keep dropping my hand down when I defend. Is that OK?
No. Trying to drop your hand down will make a slower defense (since the hand is up and the punch is going down), and will leave your face open to additional punches.

I lead with my elbow, but the punch still comes very close to my body. What is wrong?
Most likely, you're defending close to your body. Reach your defense forward by extending from the upper arm and shoulder (similar to the way in which a regular Inside Defense travels forward and inward).

Training Tips: When practicing with a partner, it's very important for the attacker to make a strong fist to protect himself. If you defend early, your elbow or forearm may block the punch instead of redirecting it, and the attacker may crack his knuckles on the hard bones of your arm. This is unpleasant. Making a fist will protect the attacker's hand from any real damage.

Note: It's always slightly more difficult to make the body defense on your strong side (i.e., on your right side if you're right-handed). Since that hip is back, it's a bit harder to turn that hip forward to blade the body the other way. Be sure to turn your right hip and shoulder far enough forward to make the body defense. Fortunately, most attackers are right-handed, which means that if you must defend on this side, you're usually defending against their weaker punch.

Remember, the body will always move more slowly than the arm—depend on the redirecting movement first, and use the body defense as insurance. Even though your body moves, let your arm and shoulder move first and be independent of your body; if you stiffen up too much, the entire technique will depend on the body movement, which will often be slower.

Be sure to tighten your abdominal muscles as you defend so that you'll be prepared to absorb the punch if it gets through. Also, contracting your abs shortens the length of your torso so that your defense (from elbow to fingers) covers more of your body.

Outside Defenses

As the name implies, Outside Defenses are made by moving the hand from an inside position outward, away from the center of the body. These defenses are made against straight punches that come from angles outside of our hands.

Defense against Straight Punch from an Outside Angle

ATTACK The attacker throws a right straight punch from the side, or from a diagonal position, or perhaps from the front if your hands are in the wrong position. Imagine having your hands up, but having an attacker standing at an angle to you. His straight punch will travel on a path outside one of your hands, rather than between them.

IMMEDIATE DANGER *Being struck.* The primary danger is being hit.

SECONDARY DANGERS *Disorientation, balance.* If the initial attack is not blocked, the defender may find himself disoriented by the first strike, or have the wind knocked out of him, or be knocked off balance, and therefore open to additional strikes.

SOLUTION *Outside Defenses 1-5*

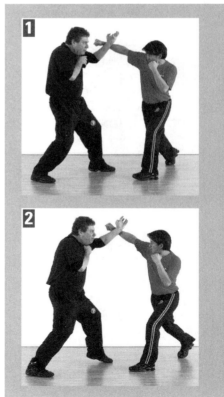

As the attack travels forward, redirect the punch with an outward movement of the closest hand (your left). There are five variations of the Outside Defense. In ALL cases, try to defend at the attacker's wrist or hand, rather than farther up the arm.

Note: For the sake of clarity, we'll assume that ALL punches are straight punches coming from your left side—either in front of you but slightly to the side, or directly from the side, as described below. For an attacker standing on the other side, simply use the other hand. Each defense works both right and left punches (with a few comments, as noted below).

1 An attacker stands slightly to your left and throws a right straight punch. Bring your forward hand up in a short arc. As your defense makes contact, rotate your wrist so that your thumb rolls toward the attacking hand. The motion of this arc MUST cross in front of your face since that's where the punch is probably going. Redirect the punch away from you while making a small body defense with your head.

2 An attacker stands slightly to your left and throws a straight punch. Bring your forward hand up in a short arc, with the back of your hand leading the motion. The motion of this arc MUST cross in front of your face since that's where the punch is probably going. Redirect the punch away from you while making a small body defense with your head.

3 An attacker stands slightly to your left and throws a straight punch. Roll your left forearm upward, rotating your forearm and wrist as you do, to redirect the punch upward. At the same time, make a body defense by contracting your abs and bending your knees slightly to drop below the punch.

4 An attacker stands slightly to your left and throws a straight punch. Stab your left hand outward, keeping your elbow down, so that your hand and arm slide along his arm, redirecting it. Keep your head tucked low but your eyes forward so that you can see the fight. Also, keep your shoulders square to the attacker. As you feel his arm being redirected, open your defending arm outward to further move the punch away from you. This is a "stabbing" defense, and is the prelude to Stick Defenses that you'll learn later on in Krav Maga.

5 An attacker stands very much to the side (note the difference from the other positions). Make a motion similar to #1 and #2, but lead with the pinky side of your hand and open your shoulder more to the side to redirect the punch away from you. Make a small body defense.

Note: Although most of these defenses work in all situations, some are preferred against certain specific attacks. For instance:

Defense #5 (leading with the pinky) is much better against attacks from the side than attacks from the front because when the pinky leads the motion, the shoulder tends to be weak until it opens up more.

Defense #4 (stabbing defense) is an excellent defense if you see the attack early and want to burst forward, defending it before it can get close to you. Also, the stabbing defense is very good against big "haymaker" punches because it allows you to burst in aggressively.

Defense #3 (rolling the arm up) is an excellent all-purpose defense, and works very well against almost all angles of attack.

Defenses #1 are #2 are very similar. Defense #1 (leading with the thumb) tends to redirect the attack more since the rotation of your wrist "rolls" the attack away from you.

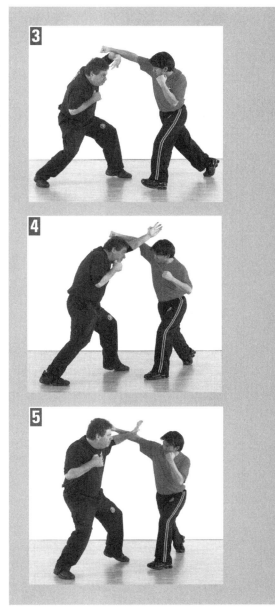

continued on next page

DEFENSES **111**

Defense against Straight Punch from an Outside Angle

continued from previous page

INITIAL COUNTERATTACK *Straight Punch (page 71).* As one hand defends, deliver a straight punch with the other hand. Any straight punch will do, but here are a few specifics for each variation of defense:

- #1 and #2 Straight punch to the face.
- #3 As your arm goes up and your body drops down slightly, send a straight punch either to the face or to the body. The face is preferred, but you may need to punch to the body if you drop low.
- #4 With the stabbing defense, you have an excellent opportunity to make a simultaneous counterattack to the face.
- #5 As the defending arm and shoulder open up, turn your body and throw a straight punch to the face.

NEUTRALIZING THE ATTACKER After the initial counterstrike, the defender should continue to attack with punches, kicks, elbows, and knees. Students must focus on rendering the attacker unwilling or unable to continue the assault.

KEY POINTS

- all the defenses are redirecting defenses
- add a body defense
- defend with the hand closest to the attack

COMMONLY ASKED QUESTIONS

Why do we have five different options? Doesn't Krav Maga try to simplify things and avoid lots of decision making?
Yes, and once you've learned all five variations, you should feel free to pick and choose which ones work best for your body. However, each variation has strengths against certain angles, as noted above, so it helps to know them all.

Would I ever use the Outside Defenses if the attacker is standing directly in front of me?
Possibly. Suppose the attacker is standing directly in front of you, but your hands are held too low. When the attacker throws a straight punch, it would take too long to bring your hand up and then make an Inside Defense. An Outside Defense is a faster option.

Would I ever use Defense #5 against an attacker who is more to the front? Do I only use it when the attacker is very much to the side?
Most people find this defense strongest against attacks from the side. However, if you feel you can make a strong defense when the attacker is more forward, you can do so.

Does it ever matter if the attacker throws a left or a right punch?
As long as you can defend near his wrist, it does not matter to the defense at all. If you defend farther up his arm, in some cases the attacker can bend his elbow and come around your defense. Of course, which punch he throws will determine whether you end up on his live or dead side. You should always counterattack aggressively to prevent him from making additional attacks.

Defense against Hook Punch

*There are two types of defenses against a Hook Punch: an "extended" defense, which we prefer, and a "covering" defense, which we use when the attacker is very close to us. The **extended defense** is very much like a 360° defense. However, there's a significant change in assumption. In this case, we assume that the defender knows he is in a fight and is not using a reflexive motion. We prefer the extended defense for street fighting because it defends the attack farther from the body; this is beneficial when weapons may be involved. However, there are times when a **covering defense** is necessary, especially in a fist fight when the attacker is very close and throwing fast punches.*

Defense against Hook Punch (Extended)

ATTACK The attacker throws a right hook punch to the head or body.

IMMEDIATE DANGER *Being struck.* The primary danger is being hit.

SECONDARY DANGERS *Disorientation, balance.* If the initial attack is not blocked, the defender may find himself disoriented by the first strike, or have the wind knocked out of him, or be knocked off balance, and therefore open to additional strikes.

SOLUTION *Hook Punch Defense*

1 As the attack comes around, block it with your forearm, keeping a 90° bend in your elbow. Make a fist and have the back of your hand face the attack. Usually, you'll send your arm out to the side in line with your shoulder, but the hook punch can come at a variety of angles, and the most important principle to keep in mind is to defend at the attacker's wrist. If you defend farther up the arm, the attack may hook around your defense. Tuck your chin and raise your shoulder to help protect your head. You can also add a small body defense by leaning your head slightly forward, inside the arc of the hook punch.

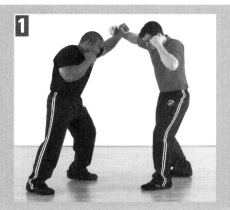

continued on next page

continued from previous page

INITIAL COUNTERATTACK *Straight Punch (page 71).* It's possible to deliver a simultaneous counterattack, although often you'll find the counterattack coming slightly after the defense. Straight punches are the most likely, but you may also try an elbow (since the attacker tends to be closer when throwing most hook punches).

NEUTRALIZING THE ATTACKER After the initial counterstrike, the defender should continue to strike to the body and face. Students must focus on rendering the attacker unwilling or unable to continue the assault.

KEY POINTS

- make a defense similar to 360, except that you make a fist and defend with the back of your hand and arm, rather than the blade
- put your weight and power behind the defense
- defend at the wrist so that the attack does not hook around your defense
- tuck your chin and raise your shoulder

COMMONLY ASKED QUESTIONS

Can't I just do a 360° defense?
Yes. The advantage of a 360 is that it's faster. However, the 360° defense assumes you are in a poor state of readiness, with hands down or at least unprepared. This defense assumes that you know you're in a fight, with your hands up in a fighting position with the pinky side of your hand forward. From this position, it may take a little longer to rotate the blade of your arm around, so the Hook Punch Defense may be preferred.

What happens if I don't defend at the wrist?
Hook punches are designed to "hook" around a defense. If you defend farther up the arm, toward the attacker's elbow, you're letting the fist come around your defense and possibly hit you.

What if the hook punch is to the body?
Follow the same principles, but you would make a defense similar to 360° Defense #4.

Training Tips: Because hook punches are powerful, be sure your defense is very strong and that you put weight behind it.

Defense against Hook Punch (Covering)

ATTACK The attacker throws a right hook punch to the head or body.

IMMEDIATE DANGER *Being struck.* The primary danger is being hit.

SECONDARY DANGERS *Disorientation, balance.* If the initial attack is not blocked, the defender may find himself disoriented by the first strike, or have the wind knocked out of him, or be knocked off balance, and therefore open to additional strikes.

SOLUTION *Hook Punch Defense (Covering)*

1 As the attack comes around to head, bring your arm up, elbow bent, so that your forearm and upper arm both cover the side of your head. Your hand should be back far enough so that your forearm/biceps makes the defense, NOT the hand. Have your hand in a fist. Keep your chin down and your arm pressed against the side of your head. Your elbow should point forward.

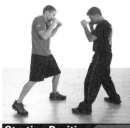

Starting Position

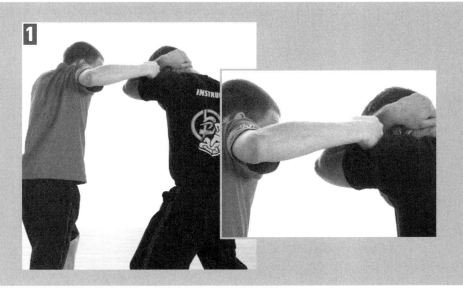

continued on next page

DEFENSES **115**

Defense against Hook Punch (Covering)

continued from previous page

INITIAL COUNTERATTACK *Straight Punch (page 71), Front Kick (page 92), or Hook Punch (page 85).*
It's not usually possible to deliver a simultaneous counterattack, since you're absorbing more of the punch. However, as soon as possible, deliver a counterattack such as a front kick to the groin, straight punch (often with the arm that just defended), or a hook punch with the free hand.

NEUTRALIZING THE ATTACKER After the initial counterstrike, the defender should continue to strike to the body and face. Students must focus on rendering the attacker unwilling or unable to continue the assault.

KEY POINTS

- bring your arm up to cover the side of the head with both the forearm and the upper arm
- your hand should be back far enough so that your forearm, not your hand, is defending
- tuck your chin and keep your arm pressed to the side of your head, elbow forward

COMMONLY ASKED QUESTIONS

When I defend, I feel my head getting jarred. What's wrong?
Keep your forearm pressed against your head more. If there is space between your arm and your head, when the hook punch hits your arm, it will bang into your head and give you a jolt. Note that this defense does absorb the strike, so you may feel some impact. However, the power should be distributed along your forearm and upper arm, reducing its effect.

Why does Krav Maga prefer the extended defense instead of this one?
The extended defense allows you to defend farther from your body, which is important in a street fight when the attacker might be holding a knife you do not see. If you use the covering defense in that case, the knife would stab into the arm, and possibly into the head. In addition, the covering defense exposes the ribs, leaving you open to body shots.

If the covering defense has these weaknesses, why teach it?
Sometimes during a fight, the attacker comes very close and throws fast hook punches. There's often no time to send the arm out and away from the body. If there were time, we'd prefer the extended defense in all cases.

Defense against Uppercut Punch

This is a redirecting defense. Although the technique is somewhat different from the Inside Defense, the redirecting principles are the same.

ATTACK The attacker throws a right uppercut punch to the head or body.

IMMEDIATE DANGER *Being struck.* The primary danger is being hit.

SECONDARY DANGERS *Disorientation, balance.* If the initial attack is not blocked, the defender may find himself disoriented by the first strike, or have the wind knocked out of him, or be knocked off balance, and therefore open to additional strikes.

SOLUTION *Uppercut Punch Defense*

1-3 As the uppercut punch rises, bring your left forearm inward and upward, redirecting the uppercut punch up and slightly to the side. The side of your arm should touch the side of the attacker's arm. As you defend, rotate your wrist—this rotation will help redirect the punch farther from your body. Keep your hand up! Your elbow should lead the motion. At the same time, make a body defense by "blading" your body to the dead side. Do NOT follow the punch up too high—keep your hands in the ready position. Defend just enough to avoid the punch.

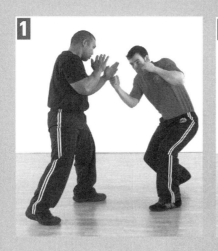
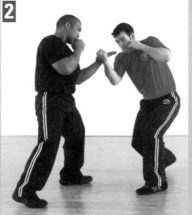
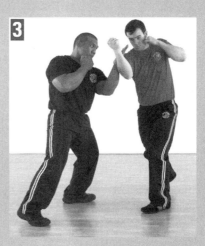

continued on next page

continued from previous page

Note the similarities to the Inside Defense against a Straight Punch Low (page 108). The mechanics are very similar, except that in most cases the uppercut punch rises, so we follow that path. Sometimes an attacker can throw an uppercut punch that travels forward (such as an uppercut punch to the body); in that case, this defense looks and feels even more like the Inside Defense against a Straight Punch Low.

INITIAL COUNTERATTACK *Straight Punch (page 71) or Hook Punch (page 85).* As you make the defense, counterattack immediately with the other hand, throwing a straight punch or a hook punch. Other counterattacks are also possible, but these will usually feel the strongest.

NEUTRALIZING THE ATTACKER After the initial counterstrike, the defender should continue to strike to the body and face. Students must focus on rendering the attacker unwilling or unable to continue the assault.

KEY POINTS

- redirect the punch by guiding it upward and away
- lead with your elbow; keep your hand up
- the principles are very similar to the Inside Defense against Straight Punch Low
- blade your body to make a body defense
- do not "follow" the punching arm up too high; defend just enough to avoid the punch

COMMONLY ASKED QUESTIONS

Why is it so important to lead with the elbow?
Leading with the elbow ensures that your hand stays up. If you think of leading with the hand, your hand may drop down. Also, since the uppercut punch starts low and travels high, if you lead with the elbow, you'll tend to redirect the punch earlier in time.

How does the wrist rotation help?
Hold your forearm up and rotate your wrist. You'll see the forearm widen slightly as the flatter part of the arm turns toward you. This width helps to redirect the punch farther away.

Sometimes when I practice, the uppercut punch is blocked by the front of my arm rather than redirected to the side. Is that OK?
This generally means that you are defending very, very early and getting your arm into the path of the attack rather than touching the side of the arm and redirecting. While this can happen in training, it's very rare that we're this early in a real fight!

Defenses against Lower Body Combatives

When defending against kicks, there are two main possibilities: using your legs or hands. When defending low kicks, it's always preferable to defend with your own legs whenever possible. This allows you to keep your hands up to defend punches, or frees your hands to counterattack immediately. However, there are occasions when this is not practical. For instance, if your legs are already damaged, the ground is slippery, or you're already doubled over after receiving a blow, your legs may be unavailable to make a defense. Under these circumstances, there is no choice but to use your hands.

Defense against Front Kick (Redirecting with Shin)

ATTACK The attacker throws a rising kick to the groin.

IMMEDIATE DANGER *Being struck (rather painfully!).* The primary danger is being hit.

SECONDARY DANGERS *Disorientation, balance.* Groin kicks are not always as bad as they appear in the movies, but they can cause a) pain that temporarily disables you and b) an instinctive reaction to scoot your hips back and pinch your knees in to protect your groin, which can compromise your balance, leaving you open to additional strikes.

SOLUTION *Leg Defense (Redirecting)*

1 As the attacking foot rises, lift your forward knee up and across the line of your groin to redirect the kick, letting it slide up and away. Your knee should lead the motion, but your foot should be almost right beneath your knee. If your knee leads too much, you'll stop the kick rather than redirect it, and this might hurt your shin. Allow the movement to redirect the kick, rather than stop it. Be sure to keep your hands up in case he follows up with punches.

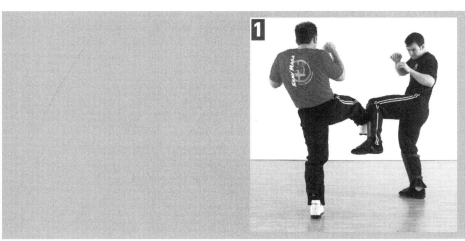

continued on next page

Defense against Front Kick (Redirecting with Shin)

continued from previous page

Note: Although this has less of the sliding action of an Inside Defense, in principle this kick defense is the same as the Inside Defense against a Straight Punch (page 106).

INITIAL COUNTERATTACK *Straight Punch (page 71).* Counterattack as soon as possible, usually with a straight punch. Although practice will help you learn which punch feels better to your body, you'll find that punching with the hand opposite from your defending leg will probably give the most power.

NEUTRALIZING THE ATTACKER After the initial counterstrike, the defender should continue to strike to the body and face. Students must focus on rendering the attacker unwilling or unable to continue the assault.

KEY POINTS

- raise your knee and leg diagonally across the line of your groin
- your knee should lead the motion, but your foot should be almost beneath your knee to avoid creating an angle against the attack
- redirect the kick, letting it slide up and away
- keep your hands up!

COMMONLY ASKED QUESTIONS

The instructions say to defend with the forward leg. Do I use that leg against either of his kicks?
Yes. You should defend any front kick to the groin with your forward leg. Whether he uses his left or right leg, the line of attack will be the same, and your forward leg can defend your groin the fastest.

If we're worried about creating an angle against the attack, why lead with the knee at all?
Because your primary concern is to protect your groin. Remember: the attacker's kick is rising. If you think of leading this motion with your foot, the kick might have risen higher than that before you react. Leading with the knee offers the most immediate protection.

I feel like I understand the defense, but I'm always late. What's wrong?
There may be several reasons you are late. First, you can work on identifying the attack. Do slow work with a partner, having him throw slow-motion kicks so you learn to identify how the kick looks as it begins. Then have your partner do slow work, mixing in straight punches and front kicks, until you learn to pick up the differences in body movements.

Another problem may be mechanical. Many beginners make this defense by "pushing off" the ground with their foot. This will slow you down because it requires your foot to be firmly set before it can push upward. A tell-tale indication of this mistake is the habit of quickly shuffling or re-adjusting your stance at the beginning of the defense. Instead of pushing off with the foot to lift your leg, think of lifting your knee from the hip (this is the work done by your hip flexors, or ilio-psoas). You don't need to know any fancy terminology—just lift your knee rather than push off the ground with your foot, and you'll find the mechanics working faster for you.

Defense against Low Round Kick (Using the Shin)

ATTACK The attacker throws a right round kick to the leg (knee or thigh).

IMMEDIATE DANGER *Knee damage, temporary dysfunction of the leg.* A round kick can hit the side of the knee, disabling it, or it can hit the side of the thigh, striking nerves in such a way as to temporarily disable the leg.

SECONDARY DANGERS *Balance.* Even if no serious damage is done, a strong low kick can shake the defender's foundation, upsetting balance and putting him at a disadvantage.

SOLUTION *Shin Block*

1 As the attack comes around to the leg, raise your left knee, with your knee forward and foot slightly back, and point it at the kick. You want to take the kick on the front of your shin, rather than the side. Your lower leg should have some tension but also a little give, like a shock absorber, to reduce the impact. Also, because many attackers chop down with their low kicks, keeping your foot back and behind your knee creates a receding angle so that a downward-sloping kick will slide down the leg. This helps minimize the shin-to-shin impact. Try to make contact with a hard part of your defense against a weak part of his attack, namely, your upper shin against his ankle. Fights are wild and full of variation, so we cannot guarantee there will be no shin-to-shin contact, but you should try to point your knee at his foot.

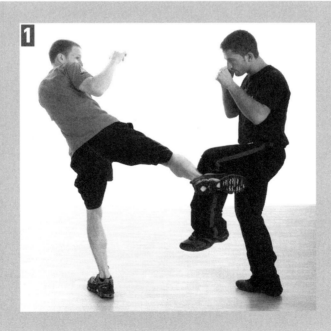

continued on next page

Defense against Low Round Kick (Using the Shin)

continued from previous page

Note: Keep your hands up! The kick may come higher than you expected. For defenses against high round kicks, please see *Complete Krav Maga*.

INITIAL COUNTERATTACK *Straight Punch (page 71) or Front Kick to the Groin (page 92).* A simple counterattack is to deliver a right straight punch as you put your foot back down after defending. Another alternative is to defend the round kick, touch your defending foot to the ground, and immediately spring up with a front kick to the attacker's groin, which will be open if he hasn't recovered quickly from his round kick.

NEUTRALIZING THE ATTACKER After the initial counterstrike, the defender should continue to strike to the body and face. Students must focus on rendering the attacker unwilling or unable to continue the assault.

KEY POINTS

- raise your knee and point it at the oncoming kick
- your lower leg should act as a shock absorber
- defend with a strong part of your defense (the thick part of the shin bone) against a weak part of the attack (the attacker's ankle)

COMMONLY ASKED QUESTIONS

When I defend, I just feel like I'm getting kicked in the shin. What's wrong?
You're making the defense too rigid. Don't build a wall—raise a shock absorber. As the kick strikes your shin, give a little so that the impact is minimized. *Note:* DON'T give too much, or the kick will sweep right through your defense.

In a real fight, won't this just hurt my shin?
It might. This is why we teach another defense (Absorbing with Thigh, described on page 123). Mixed martial arts and Muay Thai fighters use this defense all the time, but many of them condition their shins to take this punishment and minimize the pain. You probably have no plans to do that! However, keep in mind that in a real fight, which usually lasts only a short time, you may only have to deal with one of these kicks. Defend it with the strong part of your shin against his ankle, "give" a little with your shin, and you should be OK.

Defense against Low Round Kick (Absorbing with Thigh)

ATTACK The attacker throws a right round kick to the leg (knee or thigh).

IMMEDIATE DANGER *Knee damage, temporary dysfunction of the leg.* A round kick can hit the side of the knee, disabling it, or it can hit the side of the thigh, striking nerves in such a way as to temporarily disable the leg.

SECONDARY DANGERS *Balance.* Even if no serious damage is done, a strong low kick can shake the defender's foundation, upsetting balance and putting him at a disadvantage.

SOLUTION *Absorbing with Thigh*

1 As the attack comes around to the leg, bend your left knee and point it at the kick, flexing your quadriceps. Absorb the kick across the front of your quads; do NOT try to absorb the kick on the side of your leg. If your reaction is early enough, lean slightly forward to absorb the kick before it reaches maximum power.

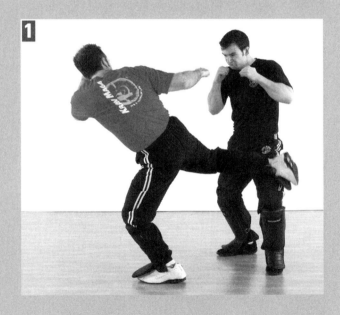

Note: Keep your hands up! The kick may come higher than you expected. For defenses against high round kicks, please see *Complete Krav Maga*.

continued on next page

Defense against Low Round Kick (Absorbing with Thigh)

continued from previous page

INITIAL COUNTERATTACK *Straight Punch (page 71).* A simple counterattack is to deliver a right straight punch. Unlike the counterattack for the Shin Block (page 121), which happens slightly after the defense, this counterattack *can* be delivered simultaneously with the absorbing defense. It's a very effective, and sometimes devastating, defense/counterattack combination against a round kick.

NEUTRALIZING THE ATTACKER After the initial counterstrike, the defender should continue to strike to the body and face. Students must focus on rendering the attacker unwilling or unable to continue the assault.

KEY POINTS

- point your knee and the top of your quadriceps at the oncoming kick while flexing your quads. Make sure your knee is bent
- absorb the kick on the front of your quads, NOT the side of the leg

COMMONLY ASKED QUESTIONS

This really hurts! What am I doing wrong?
Possibly nothing. This is an absorbing defense. You are, in fact, taking the kick, but you're just trying to do it in a way that limits damage and disburses the force. However, it's possible that you can reduce the impact by leaning in and catching the kick before it reaches full power. Also, be sure that you are absorbing the kick on the front of your quads, not the side. Absorbing the kick on the side of your leg, where a sensitive nerve can be struck, causes a great deal of pain.

I was told that I can build up the muscle if I keep practicing this absorbing technique. Is that true?
You should definitely practice this absorbing technique, but it won't build your muscles. Muscles do not get stronger when you hit them repeatedly. Practicing will help by improving your ability to flex the quadriceps, and to time the moment of flexion as you absorb. Plus, you get used to the pain, and it therefore seems to diminish.

Hand Defense against Groin Kick (Reflexive)

ATTACK The attacker throws a rising right kick to the groin when you're totally unprepared and in a neutral stance.

IMMEDIATE DANGER *Being struck (rather painfully!).* The primary danger is being hit.

SECONDARY DANGERS *Disorientation, balance.* Groin kicks are not always as bad as they appear in the movies, but they can cause a) pain that temporarily disables you and b) an instinctive reaction to put your hands down, scoot your hips back, and pinch your knees in to protect your groin, which can compromise your balance, leaving you open to additional strikes.

SOLUTION *Reflexive Defense against Front Kick*

1 As the attack rises, bend at the waist and reach down to sweep your left arm diagonally forward and across the line of your groin. Simultaneously bring your right hand up and across your face so that it can defend either a right or left punch. The defending arm should be straight (like a 2x4 from fingertips to shoulder; do NOT bend your wrist, although you can keep a slight bend in your elbow to avoid hyperextension. You can use any part of your arm to defend, but the higher up your arm the kick rises, the closer it comes to your body. The sweeping hand should redirect the kick away from your body. Make a body defense by blading your body, with the defending-side shoulder and hip moving forward.

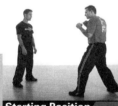
Starting Position

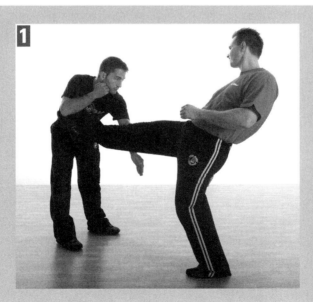

continued on next page

Hand Defense against Groin Kick (Reflexive)

continued from previous page

INITIAL COUNTERATTACK

Straight Punch. As you make the defense, burst in and trap the attacker's arm with the non-defending hand (for most people, this will be their right hand). Switch hands so that your left is trapping the attacker's arm, and counterattack with your right. Alternately, you can use your right hand to trap the attacker's arm and counterattack with your left hand. This is faster, but usually less powerful.

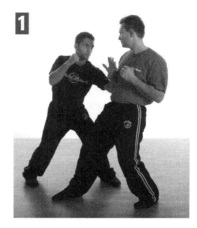
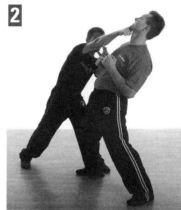

NEUTRALIZING THE ATTACKER

After the initial counterstrike, the defender should continue to strike to the body and face. Students must focus on rendering the attacker unwilling or unable to continue the assault.

KEY POINTS

- reach down and sweep your defending arm diagonally forward and across the line of your groin to redirect the kick
- blade your body—defending side forward—as a body defense
- bring your other hand up and across your face to protect against punches
- keep your defending arm straight from fingertips to shoulder (you may keep a small bend in your elbow to avoid hyperextension)

COMMONLY ASKED QUESTIONS

Can I use the same hand to defend either kick?
Yes. As with the Defense against Front Kick (page 119), the line of attack is the same with either kick, so you can use the same arm against either kick. This is helpful because of a basic assumption: We assume that we're totally unprepared for this attack, and we're standing in a neutral position. If this is true, there's no time to recognize which kick is coming at us, so we must simply defend as soon as possible. Depending on the kick the attacker uses, you may end up on the live side and open to his additional attacks. This is why you must counterattack immediately and aggressively.

Why do we assume we are so late in doing this defense?
Although it works, this is not our most effective or comfortable defense. However, from a position of extreme disadvantage, reacting on instinct, this defense is closest to our body's reflexive reactions (hands going down, hips going back).

Training Tips: Reach down so that you can defend the kick as early as possible. Reach slightly forward so that, if you're fairly early, you can defend at the knee before the foot starts to rise.

Hand Defense against Groin Kick (Stabbing)

ATTACK The attacker throws a rising right kick to the groin when you're in a fighting stance.

IMMEDIATE DANGER *Being struck (rather painfully!).* The primary danger is being hit.

SECONDARY DANGERS *Disorientation, balance.* Groin kicks are not always as bad as they appear in the movies, but they can cause a) pain that temporarily disables you and b) an instinctive reaction to put your hands down, scoot your hips back, and pinch your knees in to protect your groin, which can compromise your balance, leaving you open to additional strikes.

SOLUTION *Outside Stabbing Defense against Front Kick*

1 As the attack rises, burst in toward the attacker on a slight diagonal angle and stab down toward the attacker's knee with your rear (right) hand. Keep your elbow in and the meaty part of your hand pointing back toward your body. This ensures that your arm is straight, creating no angle against the kick. Keep your shoulders square to your attacker—turning your right side (the defending arm) forward will redirect the kick into your body, not away from it. Be sure your left hand is up, protecting your face, in case the kick is followed by an immediate punch. As soon as you feel the kick sliding along your arm, move the arm slightly outward, creating a larger defense.

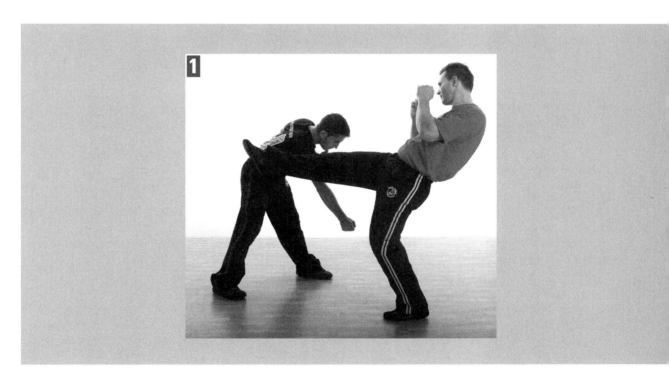

continued on next page

INITIAL COUNTERATTACK *Straight Punch.* As you make the defense, burst in and trap the attacker's arm with the non-defending hand (for most people, this will be the left hand) and deliver a counterattack with your right. Alternately, you can throw an immediate (even simultaneous) counterattack with your left hand. This is a much faster, but most likely weaker, counter.

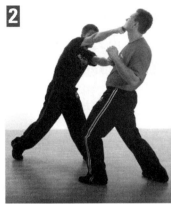
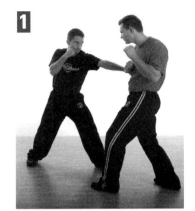

NEUTRALIZING THE ATTACKER
After the initial counterstrike, the defender should continue to strike to the body and face. Students must focus on rendering the attacker unwilling or unable to continue the assault.

KEY POINTS

- stab your rear hand downward, elbow in and down, to redirect the kick
- burst in as you defend
- keep your shoulders square so that the kick is redirected off your body
- keep your other hand up and slightly forward to protect your face

COMMONLY ASKED QUESTIONS

Should I always use my rear hand to make this defense?
Yes. The kick is redirected off your body. Using the rear hand means that the kick is redirecting toward the rear hip as well. Because that hip is back, there is space for the kick to travel through and then off the body. If you try to defend with the forward hand, your forward hip may be in the way, and you may take the kick on your body.

Is this defense better than the reflexive defense?
The stabbing action is stronger, and redirects the kick with a simpler motion. Basically, by stabbing, you are building a ramp that simply guides the kick away. In most cases, once you stab to the inside of the leg and the leg begins to slide up your arm, the kick is automatically redirected. The "sweeping" action of the reflexive defense works well, but isn't quite so absolute.

Hand Defense against Front Kick to the Face

ATTACK The attacker throws a right rising kick to your face.

IMMEDIATE DANGER *Being struck.* The primary danger is being hit in the face.

SECONDARY DANGERS *Disorientation, balance.* Whether or not you actually take the kick, the attack may cause you to lean back, robbing you of balance and initiative.

SOLUTION *Inside Defense against High Front Kick*

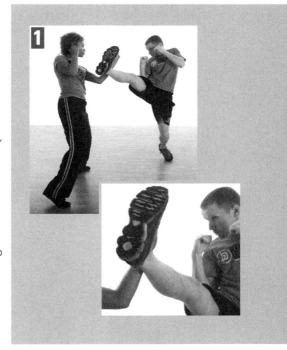

1 As the kick rises, bring your forward (left) arm across your face and upper body, parallel to the floor. Your hand may be in a fist—rotate it so that the meaty part of your hand makes the deflection. As you make the hand defense, add a small body defense by blading your body with the left side forward. Be sure your weight stays in the fight! Keep your hand up and your elbow inward so that your forearm is vertical. If you dip your hand down, you'll make an angle against the attack and get kicked in the arm.

INITIAL COUNTERATTACK *Straight Punch.* Immediately counterattack, most often with a right straight punch.

NEUTRALIZING THE ATTACKER After the initial counterstrike, the defender should continue to strike to the body and face. Students must focus on rendering the attacker unwilling or unable to continue the assault.

KEY POINTS

- redirect the kick with the forearm of your forward hand
- blade your body to make a body defense
- don't lean back; stay in the fight!

COMMONLY ASKED QUESTIONS

Should I always defend with my forward hand against either kick?
Yes. The line of attack is the same. Be aware that you may end up on the live side. Always counterattack aggressively and decisively.

I keep getting kicked in the arm. What's wrong?
You're probably defending by dropping your hand down. This usually results in a kick on your forearm. Redirect the kick by moving your forearm (hand up, elbow down) across your body.

Is it better to make a fist or leave your hand open?
An open hand will be more relaxed, and therefore faster. A closed fist will tense the muscles of the forearm and protect them in case your timing is off and you absorb any power from the kick. Therefore, both have pros and cons. Ideally, an open hand results in a faster defense.

Hand Defense against Knee Strike

ATTACK The attacker throws a right knee to the groin, midsection, or face.

IMMEDIATE DANGER *Being struck.* The primary danger is being hit.

SECONDARY DANGERS *Additional counterattacks, takedowns.* Because knees happen in close situations, the attacker is very close to you. If the first knee does damage, you may be open to a number of additional strikes and other attacks.

SOLUTION *Forearm Block (like 360°)*

1 As the knee rises, make a 360° defense against the middle of the thigh with the arm closest to the attacking limb (generally the left arm). Preferably, you should defend relatively early—the more momentum the knee builds up, the more impact you'll feel when defending. Be aggressive—attack the leg as it rises, rather than waiting for it.

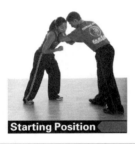

Starting Position

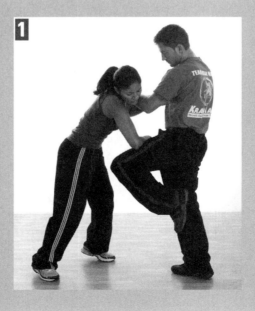

INITIAL COUNTERATTACK *Punch to the groin (page 75).* As you make the defense, strike to the groin with an uppercut punch or open-hand strike.

NEUTRALIZING THE ATTACKER After the initial counterstrike, the defender should disengage from any hold the attacker may have, and continue to strike to the body and face. Students must focus on rendering the attacker unwilling or unable to continue the assault.

KEY POINTS

- make a 360° defense—be sure to follow all the basic 360° principles, including using the blade of your arm and attacking the attack

COMMONLY ASKED QUESTIONS

Won't this defense hurt my arm?
Only if you think defensively and wait for the knee to reach your arm. Be aggressive and defend the attack before it develops full power.

What if I cannot disengage from his hold?
Continue with counterattacks and prepare to defend again. You're in an undesirable position, but he is open to attacks if you punch to his groin and midsection.

Defenses against Holds, Grabs, and Chokes

This section deals with chokes, headlocks, and bearhugs from a variety of positions.

Choke from the Front (Two-Handed Pluck)

ATTACK This attack happens to the defender's live side, and the attacker places both hands on the throat. The defender should train from a neutral position. Emphasis must be placed on the defender lifting the attacker's hands prior to sliding the attacker's hands outward.

Safety in training note: Do not "punch" the hands into the defender's throat when training.

IMMEDIATE DANGER *Thumbs on throat.* The primary danger in this attack is the potential of the thumbs crushing the windpipe. Without the thumbs, the attack is much less dangerous.

SECONDARY DANGERS *Balance, headbutt.* In the attack and the subsequent defense, disruption of balance and headbutts (incidental or intentional) are possible. If the defense is performed properly, these peripheral dangers should be mitigated or removed altogether.

SOLUTION *Two-Handed Pluck*

The natural reaction to this attack is to bring the hands to where the danger or pain is. The plucking motion turns this instinct into a defense, which relies on explosiveness (speed), as opposed to strength.

1 Create hooks with your hands by bringing your fingers and thumb together tightly and curling them slightly. Bring your hands up and over the attacker's hands, reaching deep inside at the point where the wrists and thumbs meet, plucking the attacker's hands up and out. This movement should be explosive from the beginning of the motion. Tuck your chin to guard against an incidental headbutt.

2 As the pluck continues parallel to your shoulders, pin the attacker's hands to your body. While this is not essential to the technique, it limits the attacker's weapons.

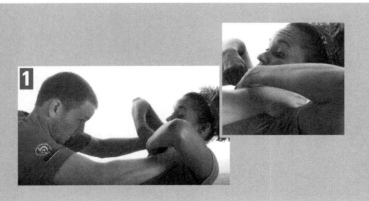

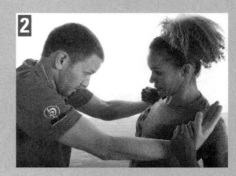

INITIAL COUNTERATTACK *Front Kick to Groin (page 92).* The front kick to the groin should be delivered as close to simultaneously to the pluck as possible. Not only will this shift the dynamics of the fight faster, but it will also mitigate the chances of an accidental headbutt. *Note:* Depending on the proximity of the attack, your knee may make contact first, but you should still throw the kick, since it may be difficult to assess the range in the moment.

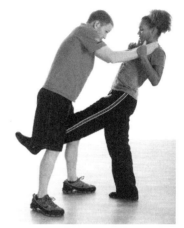

NEUTRALIZING THE ATTACKER Typical follow-ups to the groin kick are knees, more front kicks, and/or hammerfists to the back of the head, though the situation will always dictate. Regardless of the combatives used, students must focus on rendering the attacker unwilling or unable to continue the assault.

KEY POINTS

- explosive pluck, deep and at the wrist and thumb
- trap attacking hands to body
- simultaneous front kick to groin
- aggressive, follow-up combatives
- disengage when deemed safe

COMMONLY ASKED QUESTIONS

Why not just kick to the groin?
While it's important to counterattack quickly, it's necessary to eliminate the immediate danger first. In this particular case, it's possible that the kick would cause the attacker to tense and increase the pressure on the choke if the pluck were not employed.

Do I have to pin the attacker's hands?
While it's not a must to pin the hands, it will serve to prevent or delay secondary attacks.

Why is the pluck better than other defenses I have seen for this attack?
The pluck is a derivation of a natural movement, so it's more likely to work under pressure. It will also work regardless of whether the arms are bent or straight, and the same motion will be utilized versus other attacks.

Training Tips: Think of the plucking action and direction like Superman ripping off his shirt. Plucking up and out is a strong action and, if performed explosively, the attacker cannot adjust in the moment.

Give this a try: Have a friend extend her arm out straight. Ask her to resist as you gradually add downward pressure and weight on the arm. Your friend will be able to offer amazing resistance to this gradual increase. Now, ask her to do the same, but this time, and without telling her, explosively slap the arm down with your hand. She will not be able to resist this action. This is the same way the pluck works.

ATTACK This attack happens to the defender's side, and the attacker places the hands on the throat and neck. The defender should train from a neutral position. The attacker should simulate a realistic attack, building in intensity as familiarity with the defense increases. One hand is positioned in front of the throat, while the other is placed on the back of the neck.

IMMEDIATE DANGER *Hands on neck and throat.* The primary danger in this attack is the pressure on the sides of the neck, which restricts the carotid arteries and potentially the windpipe, depending on the position of the hand choking in front.

SECONDARY DANGERS *Headbutt.* After the initial defense, an incidental headbutt is possible. If the defense is performed properly, this danger should be mitigated or removed altogether.

SOLUTION *One-Hand Pluck*

1 Creating the same hook with your hand as in the front choke defense, this time using only the hand furthest from the attacker, reach up and beyond the attacker's hand.

2 In order be as explosive as possible, pluck where the wrist and thumb meet in a diagonal motion downward across your chest. To guard against an incidental headbutt, turn your head towards the attacker while simultaneously tucking your chin, exposing the top of your head to the attacker, not your face or the side of your head. As the pluck continues along your chest, pin the attacker's hand to your body. While this is not essential to the technique, it limits the attacker's weapons.

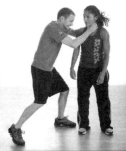
Starting Position

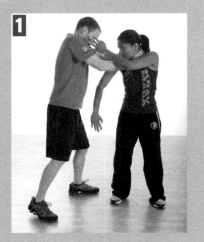

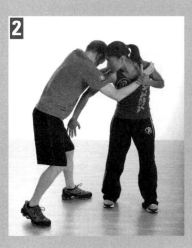

INITIAL COUNTERATTACK *Strike to Groin.* The strike to the groin should be delivered as close to simultaneously to the pluck as possible. The preferred strike is an open-hand slap because of the increased surface area it offers, but other strikes (such as hammerfist, page 88) are acceptable.

NEUTRALIZING THE ATTACKER Typical follow-ups to the groin strike are elbows to the face and head (hammerfists are also an option, if the attacker begins to move away from the strikes). The defender should continue to strike while turning to face the attacker, which will allow the defender to transition to a more advantageous fighting position. Once this position is obtained, further combatives, such as knees and kicks, may be used more readily. Regardless of the combatives used, students must focus on rendering the attacker unwilling or unable to continue the assault.

KEY POINTS

- explosive pluck, diagonally across the chest
- trap the plucked hand to body
- simultaneous strike to groin
- aggressive, follow-up combatives while turning to engage attacker
- disengage when deemed safe

COMMONLY ASKED QUESTIONS

Why would anyone attack this way?
While it's certainly possible to attack in this manner, it's also possible that the defender's initial reaction to such a threat from the front is to turn the head and upper body away, creating a choke from the side (even if the intent was to choke from the front).

Do I have to pin the attacker's hand?
While it's not a must to pin the hand, it will serve to prevent or delay secondary attacks. It's also a good training habit, since keeping the hand tight will make for a stronger pluck.

Can I go for the elbow immediately, instead of the groin strike?
Absolutely! As a matter of fact, if your hands happen to be up when the attack happens, this is probably a better option, but it's still important to strike simultaneously to the defense.

Training Tips: In order to make the pluck as successful as possible, reach beyond the attacker's hands, as if you're trying to touch your ear. Keep your hand and the defender's hand tight to your body. This action will allow you to maximize both power in the pluck and control of the attacker.

Be aware that it's very common for students to step away while making this defense and counter. This will work against the defense, since it moves towards the strength of the attack (the four fingers). Stepping away will also diminish the power of the counter and perhaps even take the defender out of range for the initial strike.

ATTACK This attack happens to the defender's dead side, and the attacker places both hands on the neck and throat. The defender should train from a neutral position. The attacker should simulate a realistic attack, building in intensity as familiarity with the defense increases.

Safety in training note: Do not "punch" the hands into the defender's neck when training, since this can cause a "whiplash" effect.

IMMEDIATE DANGER *Fingers on throat.* The primary danger in this attack is the potential of the fingers crushing the windpipe.

SECONDARY DANGERS *Balance, strikes.* In the initial defense, it's possible to be exposed to an increased risk of tripping or being swept to the ground. The defender should also be aware of the potential for strikes from the attacker.

SOLUTION *Two-Hand Pluck*

1-3 Send your hands as far back as you can, plucking the attacker's hands straight down, bringing your elbows to your sides. As your hands begin to move, tuck your chin and round your shoulders (you may find this happening instinctively). This pluck, like the others discussed, should be explosive and performed as close to the thumb and wrist of the attacker's hands as possible. While performing the pluck, step back diagonally, moving both feet.

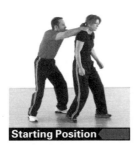

Starting Position

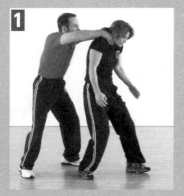

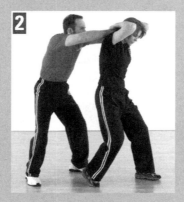

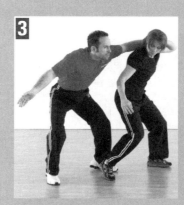

INITIAL COUNTERATTACK *Strike to Groin.* While not simultaneous, this strike should occur as a natural continuation of the plucking motion, using a slap or hammerfist to the groin. Making the diagonal step mentioned above will not only help reduce the chance of being tripped or swept, it will also line up the attacker's groin for this strike.

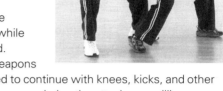

NEUTRALIZING THE ATTACKER After the initial counterstrike, the defender should continue to strike with elbows to the body and face while turning to face the attacker, still controlling the attacker's outside hand. Depending on the attacker's reaction to these strikes, longer-range weapons such as hammerfists may be employed, and the hand may be released to continue with knees, kicks, and other combatives. Regardless of the combatives used, students must focus on rendering the attacker unwilling or unable to continue the assault.

KEY POINTS

- explosive pluck at the wrist and thumb, straight down
- diagonal step to open up the groin, establish a good base, and move away from the attacker's free arm
- strike to groin, continuing the plucking motion
- aggressive, follow-up combatives while turning to engage the attacker
- disengage

COMMONLY ASKED QUESTIONS

I thought Krav Maga used simultaneous counterattacks?
While this is preferred, it's not always possible. In this case, the attack is to the defender's dead side, so strong counters are not available in tandem with the defense. The groin strike should still be made as soon as the immediate threat is addressed.

Do I have to control the attacker's hand?
While it's not a must to control the hand, it will serve to prevent or delay secondary attacks, and it aids in keeping the attacker close for follow-up counters.

If I don't continue the plucking motion to the groin, what else can I do?
This is not really much of a problem; simply transition immediately to elbows to the face, continuing to strike as you turn.

Does it matter which side I move to when making the initial defense?
From a technique standpoint, it makes no difference. However, there may be some tactical considerations that dictate moving one way or another (e.g., obstructions to one side, carrying of weapons, injuries, etc.).

Training Tips: When turning to engage the attacker, it's essential to continue striking while maintaining your footing.

In order to engage while reducing the chance of tripping on the attacker's foot, your inside foot should make a "C" on the floor as you turn, maneuvering around the attacker's foot and putting you in a fighting stance.

ATTACK This attack happens to the defender's live side, and the attacker places both hands on the throat while pushing backward. The defender should train from a neutral position and should be pushed slightly off balance. The attacker should simulate a realistic attack, building in intensity as familiarity with the defense increases.

Safety in training note: Do not "punch" the hands into the defender's throat when training. Apply the choke, then the push, to minimize the risk of injury.

IMMEDIATE DANGER *Thumbs on throat, balance.* The primary danger in this attack is the potential of the thumbs crushing the windpipe, as well as being pushed off balance.

SECONDARY DANGERS *Immediate environment.* Depending on the actual intent of the attack, the defender may be pushed into a wall, car, or other obstruction, further complicating the defense and increasing the danger. If the defense is performed early enough, this danger should be mitigated or removed altogether.

SOLUTION Rotational Defense (*note:* the defense can be made to either side, but for demonstrative purposes, sides have been designated)

The natural reaction to this attack is for the arms to go up and for the defender to step back. Both of these motions are instinctual reactions designed to maintain balance, but the technique only requires one arm.

1 As you step back with your left foot, stab your right arm straight up in the air, with the biceps and shoulder as close to your right ear as possible.

2 Turn sharply to the left, creating pressure on the attacker's wrist and relieving pressure on your throat.

3 Drop your right elbow straight down for a downward vertical strike (elbow #7) in order to clear the hands, and trap the arms using your left hand.

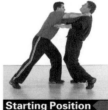
Starting Position

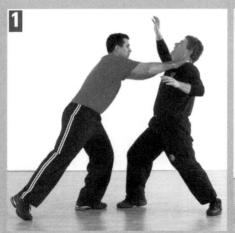
1

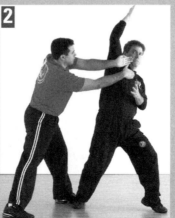
2

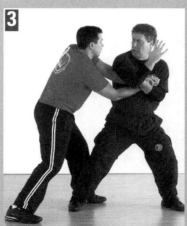
3

INITIAL COUNTERATTACK *Sideways Elbow Strike (Elbow #2) (page 79).* While not simultaneous to the defense, this elbow should immediately follow the clearing and trapping motions. Be sure to tuck your chin while delivering the elbow, and shift your weight into the counter.

NEUTRALIZING THE ATTACKER After the initial counterstrike, the defender should continue to strike with elbows and hammerfists to the head, while turning to face the attacker. Regardless of the combatives used, students must focus on rendering the attacker unwilling or unable to continue the assault.

KEY POINTS

- when training, lean back to simulate being off balance
- arm stabs straight up to defend at the wrist
- turn sharply after stepping and stabbing
- put weight into initial counter from the side
- aggressive, follow-up combatives
- disengage when deemed safe

COMMONLY ASKED QUESTIONS

This defense feels really strong. Can I do it if there is no push?
Yes, this defense is very strong, and it will certainly work against a "static" choke. Krav Maga teaches the plucking defense first, since it's more instinctual and generally takes less time to learn.

Can I defend to either side?
You should train both sides after you have developed some familiarity with the defense. The defense works whether you step with the right foot and stab with the left or vice versa.

Training Tips: Allow the "attacker" to put you off balance before making the initial step. This will help to simulate a surprise attack, and you may even start with your eyes closed to force you to defend "late."

Remember, the sharp turn makes the defense, not the elbow. It's very important to stab the arm straight up and turn your body explosively. The technique does not rely on strength, but leverage.

ATTACK This attack happens to the defender's dead side, and the attacker places both hands on the throat and neck while pushing forward. The defender should train from a neutral position and should be pushed slightly off balance. The attacker should simulate a realistic attack, building in intensity as familiarity with the defense increases.

Safety in training note: Do not "punch" the hands into the defender's neck when training. Apply the choke, then the push, to minimize the risk of injury.

IMMEDIATE DANGER *Neck, throat, balance.* The primary dangers in this attack are the potential of a whiplash effect to the neck, the fingers crushing the windpipe, and being pushed off balance.

SECONDARY DANGERS *Immediate environment.* Depending on the actual intent of the attack, the defender may be pushed into a wall, car, or other obstruction, further complicating the defense and increasing the danger. If the defense is performed early enough, this danger should be mitigated or removed altogether.

SOLUTION *Rotational Defense* (*note*: the defense can be made to either side, but for demonstrative purposes, sides have been designated)

The natural reaction to this attack is for the arms to go out and for the defender to step. Both of these motions are instinctual reactions designed to maintain balance, but the technique only requires one arm.

1 As you step forward with your right foot, stab your left arm straight forward, with the biceps and shoulder as close to the left ear as possible. Turn sharply to the left, creating pressure on the attacker's wrist and relieving pressure on your throat and neck. This turn should be greater than 90° in order to face the attacker.

2 Continue to turn, stepping back with your left foot, establishing a strong base. Drop your left elbow down to clear and trap the attacker's hands.

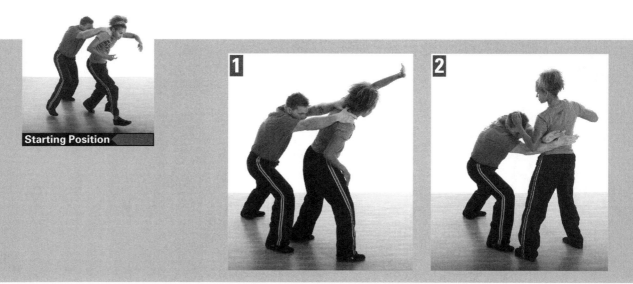

Starting Position

INITIAL COUNTERATTACK *Punch (page 71).* While not simultaneous to the defense, this punch should immediately follow the clearing and trapping motions. In keeping with the description above, this would be a right punch to the attacker's face.

NEUTRALIZING THE ATTACKER After the initial counterstrike, the defender should continue to strike with knees. Regardless of the combatives used, students must focus on rendering the attacker unwilling or unable to continue the assault.

KEY POINTS

- when training, lean forward to simulate being off balance
- arm stabs straight forward to defend at the wrist
- turn sharply after stepping and stabbing
- aggressive, follow-up combatives
- disengage when deemed safe

COMMONLY ASKED QUESTIONS

During training, my partner often goes right by me when I make the defense. What am I doing wrong?
It's very likely that you're doing nothing wrong. If the push is very strong, it's not only possible, but probable, that the attacker's momentum will carry him beyond you, which is why the step back is important.

Can I defend to either side?
You should train both sides after you have developed some familiarity with the defense. The defense works whether you step with the right foot and stab with the left or vice versa.

Is it okay to wrap the arms after clearing them?
Krav Maga prefers to teach techniques that work for everyone. By wrapping, you give some measure of control to the attacker, and if the attacker is much larger or a better grappler, this can be very problematic. By simply pinning the hands with your elbow, you have the freedom of a quick release if needed.

Training Tips: Though often a safety issue in training, it's possible to strike with the elbow and/or hammerfist of the clearing arm. This is a faster counter, but it's a difficult to train without actually striking your training partner.

In order to make the rotation easier and more effective, be sure to turn in place, as opposed to moving your shoulder backward. Such a motion will create more resistance, making the defense harder to perform.

ATTACK This is the typical "schoolyard" headlock, where the attacker wraps his arm around your head and neck. The defender should train from a neutral position. The attacker should simulate a realistic attack, building in intensity as familiarity with the defense increases.

Safety in training note: Warm up your neck before training this attack and defense.

IMMEDIATE DANGER *Balance, pressure on the neck and throat.* The primary dangers in this attack are the potential of being taken to the ground and of the forearm restricting blood flow to the brain or crushing the windpipe.

SECONDARY DANGERS *Punches.* The attacker's intent may be to hold the defender and punch to the face. If the defense is performed properly, this peripheral danger should be mitigated or removed altogether.

SOLUTION *High and Low Defense.* The natural reaction to this attack is to step to avoid falling or being taken to the ground. The arms are also likely to swing in order to aid in maintaining balance. Do not fight this natural inclination.

1 As the attack develops, step with it, turning your chin towards the attacker's hands, and tucking it in to provide a defense against punches and reduce the effects of a choke or strangulation. At the same time, your outside hand should swing low to the attacker's groin, and your inside hand should go high between your head and the attacker's head.

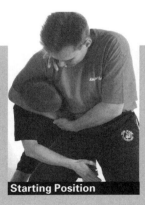

Starting Position

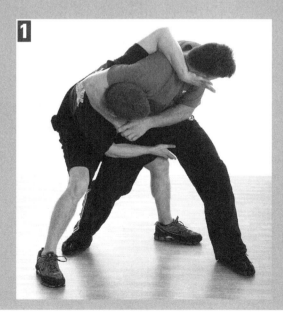

INITIAL COUNTERATTACK *Strike to Groin, Grab to Face.* The outside hand should slap or punch the groin as you're making the defense. The inside hand, placed between your head and the attacker's, should go to the attacker's face, with your thumb under the chin and index finger under the nose, avoiding the mouth.

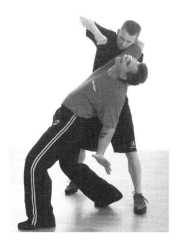

NEUTRALIZING THE ATTACKER Lift the attacker's chin and drive the attacker's head straight down, while standing up with your legs and straightening your back. Continue to use hammerfists, palm heels, and punches to the face and throat while driving the attacker down towards the ground.

KEY POINTS

- go with the pull…do not resist it
- turn and tuck your chin to minimize the chance of being punched or choked
- simultaneously strike to groin and grab to face
- once the attacker's chin is up, drive your elbow (and the attacker's head) down
- do not follow the attacker to the ground while delivering counters
- aggressive, follow-up combatives
- disengage when deemed safe

COMMONLY ASKED QUESTIONS

What if I can't get to the attacker's face?
If the attacker has hair, make a grab at the hairline, pulling the head straight back and down, continuing with combatives. It's also possible to grab the muscle on the side of the attacker's neck and twist it to induce pain and create the needed leverage. In either case, you should still make the same motion with your elbow going down along the attacker's back.

Training Tips: It's very common for students to pull the elbow out instead of down. This will not allow for the kind of leverage and control needed to make the defense and deliver multiple counters. Think of turning the attacker's head back, making a "question mark" with your hand, arm, and elbow. After this motion, take your elbow straight down, keeping the attacker in one place, not rotating and pushing him away from you.

Don't stop once you've created leverage on the neck and stood upright. Continue applying pressure to the neck and delivering combatives until the attacker is driven to the ground or taken off balance.

ATTACK With the rear headlock, the attacker wraps his arm around the neck, attacking the front of the throat or sides of the neck. The defender should train from a neutral position. The attacker should simulate a realistic attack, building in intensity as familiarity with the defense increases. It's important to note the inherent danger in this attack. Respond as early as possible to prevent a strong headlock from being applied.

Safety in training notes: Warm up your neck before training this attack and defense. Be careful not to apply too much pressure to the front of the throat. The attacker should also be aware of the potential for eye gouges.

IMMEDIATE DANGER *Crushing of the windpipe or restriction of blood flow.* In this attack, the immediate danger varies by the placement of the attacker's arm. If the forearm lies across the throat, the windpipe is in danger of being crushed. If the forearm wraps around to the other side of the neck, with the crook of the elbow at the defender's throat, the danger becomes losing consciousness as a result of the carotid arteries being restricted.

SECONDARY DANGERS *Balance.* In order to apply this headlock, it may be necessary or expedient for the attacker to pull the defender backward, compromising balance.

SOLUTION *Plucking*

The natural reaction to this attack is to bring the hands to where the danger or pain is. The plucking motion turns this instinct into a defense, which relies on explosiveness (speed) as opposed to strength. If possible, turn your chin towards the attacker's hands while tucking it down against your body.

1 Send both hands up and back towards the attacker's hands.

2 Pluck down explosively, 90° to the attack. If the attack is on the throat, this will mean along the chest. If the attack is on the sides of the neck, the pluck motion will be along the shoulder.

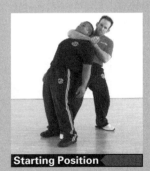
Starting Position

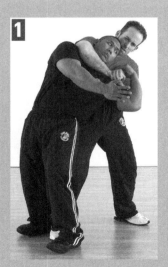

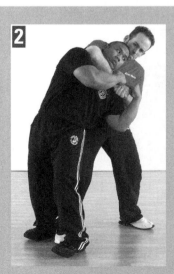

3-5 Continue to turn towards the opening created by the pluck and slide your head out immediately.

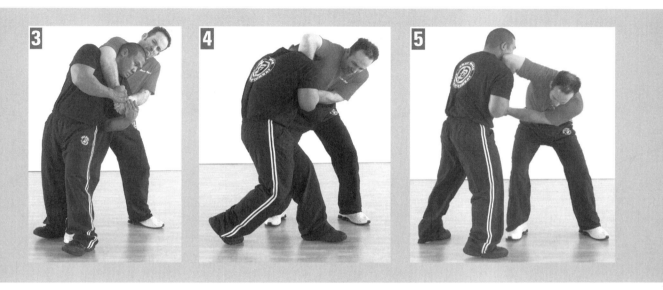

INITIAL COUNTERATTACK *Shoulder Strike.* Your inside shoulder should turn sharply into the attacker's body, creating more space in order to make it easier to remove your head from the hold.

NEUTRALIZING THE ATTACKER As soon as your head has been removed from the hold, immediately attack with knees, punches, hammerfists, or other available combatives.

KEY POINTS

- turn and tuck your chin as soon as possible
- pluck explosively, 90° to the attack
- send both hands back as far as possible
- after turning sharply with your shoulder, remove your head
- attack aggressively with whatever strikes are available

COMMONLY ASKED QUESTIONS

I'm not breaking the attacker's grip. What am I doing wrong?
It's possible that nothing is wrong with the defense. The plucking motion is designed to weaken the grip and eliminate pressure by creating space. It's not designed to break the grip, although it's attacking the attack's weakest point.

continued on next page

continued from previous page

Why can't I get my head out after making the pluck?

While you don't need much space, it's important to make sure that you're turning your chin, removing your head in such a way that it's narrower. Also, depending on the strength of the attacker, a strong and explosive shoulder turn should help to create additional space.

Training Tips: While it's important to train from positions of disadvantage, this attack is extremely dangerous and difficult to defend if very late. You should place great emphasis on defending EARLY.

In order to make the pluck as explosive as possible, think about sending the hands back, as if trying to strike the attacker's eyes, then plucking down. In most cases, going straight to the hands will not provide the momentum needed.

Bearhug from the Front with Arms Caught (No Space)

ATTACK In this attack, the defender has been grabbed around the body, from the front, with the defender's arms trapped against the body.

IMMEDIATE DANGER *None.* Unlike most other attacks, the bearhug itself does not cause damage. The actual hold presents no immediate danger.

SECONDARY DANGERS *Location change, takedown, multiple attackers.* As a hold, the danger lies in the attacker's motivation: picking up the defender to change locations, taking the defender to the ground, holding the defender in place for another attacker, etc.

SOLUTION & INITIAL COUNTERATTACK *Base and Space, Counterattack.*

1 Drop your weight immediately in order to make it more difficult for the attacker to lift you. Strike or grab the attacker's groin, with one or both hands, in order to create space.

2-3 Send the heels of your palms to your attacker's hips in order to maintain space; attack with knees to the groin and/or midsection.

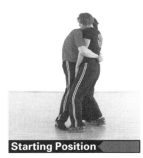

Starting Position

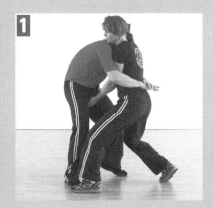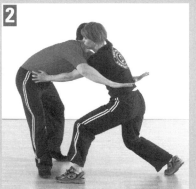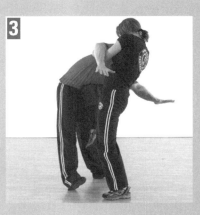

continued on next page

Bearhug from the Front with Arms Caught (No Space)

continued from previous page

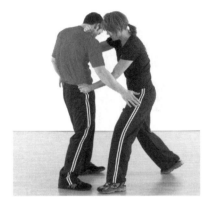

NEUTRALIZING THE ATTACKER As soon as enough space is created, control the attacker by bringing your inside arm up, grabbing where the attacker's shoulder and neck meet, laying your forearm along the attacker's neck and down his chest. This position will allow you to deliver more knees and kicks, as well as more readily defend takedown attempts.

KEY POINTS

- base and space and send counterattacks immediately
- if there is no space, create it by striking or grabbing the groin
- control the hips to maintain space
- transition control to the attacker's shoulder and neck when possible
- attack aggressively with knees and kicks
- disengage when deemed safe

COMMONLY ASKED QUESTIONS

What if there is space initially? Do I need to do the groin strike?
No, though you should begin counterattacking immediately, whether you strike the groin, stomp the foot, or whatever else is available.

With no space, I'm having a hard time accessing the groin. What is wrong?
It may be difficult to get to the groin, but if you shift your hips to one side, that should allow an avenue for attacks to the groin.

My training partner does not react very much to the initial groin strike. Is that okay?
A big reaction should not be expected, and it's not necessary. The groin strike is not expected to end the fight. If your opponent shifts his hips back slightly, just enough for you to establish a base with your feet, that is enough.

Training Tips: Remember, it may not be necessary to create space. Regardless, you should counterattack as soon as possible. Unlike other attacks, the counterattack can be first, since the hold itself is not dangerous.

When striking the groin to create space, the hands are typically quickest, but you may also strike with your knee by taking your leg back and bringing your knee in towards the groin.

Bearhug from the Front with Arms Free

ATTACK In this attack, the defender has been grabbed around the body, from the front, with the defender's arms free to move.

IMMEDIATE DANGER *None.* Unlike most other attacks, the bearhug itself does not cause damage. The actual hold presents no immediate danger.

SECONDARY DANGERS *Location change, takedown, multiple attackers.* As a hold, the danger lies in the attacker's motivation: picking up the defender to change locations, taking the defender to the ground, holding the defender in place for another attacker, etc.

SOLUTION & INITIAL COUNTERATTACK *Base and Space, Counterattack*

1 Drop your weight immediately in order to make it more difficult for the attacker to lift you; send your hips and feet back as far as possible while sending your hands to the attacker's hips.

2 Deliver knees to the groin and midsection immediately.

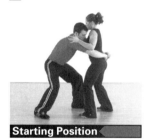

Starting Position

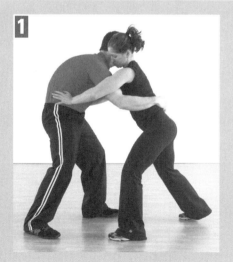

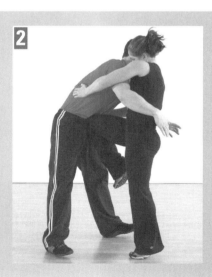

continued on next page

Bearhug from the Front with Arms Free

continued from previous page

NEUTRALIZING THE ATTACKER As soon as you can safely do so, release the attacker's hips and continue attacking. Disengage when safely possible.

KEY POINTS

- base and space and send counterattacks immediately
- control the hips to maintain space
- transition away from the attacker's hips as soon as appropriate
- attack aggressively with knees, kicks, and other combatives
- disengage when deemed safe

COMMONLY ASKED QUESTIONS

What if I can't reach around the attacker's arms to the hips?
This may be a problem if the attacker is rather large, but since there is space, you should be able to use knee strikes to aid in maintaining space and doing damage to the attacker.

Training Tips: Because of the nature of this attack, the defender is very susceptible to takedowns. It's important to send the hips and feet back explosively and counterattack with knees immediately.

For another option, see the next technique, which will also work against larger attackers who have eliminated space.

Bearhug from the Front with Arms Free (Leverage on the Neck)

ATTACK In this attack, the defender has been grabbed around the body, from the front, with the defender's arms free to move.

IMMEDIATE DANGER *None.* Unlike most other attacks, the bearhug itself does not cause damage. The actual hold presents no immediate danger.

SECONDARY DANGERS *Location change, takedown, multiple attackers.* As a hold, the danger lies in the attacker's motivation: picking up the defender to change locations, taking the defender to the ground, holding the defender in place for another attacker, etc.

SOLUTION & INITIAL COUNTERATTACK *Base and Space, Counterattack by applying leverage on the attacker's neck*

1 In order to make it more difficult for the attacker to lift you, drop your weight immediately by sending your hips and feet as far back as possible. Note that because there is no space between you, your back may be arched, making it difficult to fully "base out." It may also be difficult to strike his groin. Establish as much of a base as you can, while attacking as follows:

2 As the attacker squeezes you in, his head will generally turn to one side or the other against your chest. With your opposite side arm, reach around the attacker's head, grabbing the hair at the temple. If the attacker has no hair, reach slightly farther and grab along the nose ridge while pressing into his eyes.

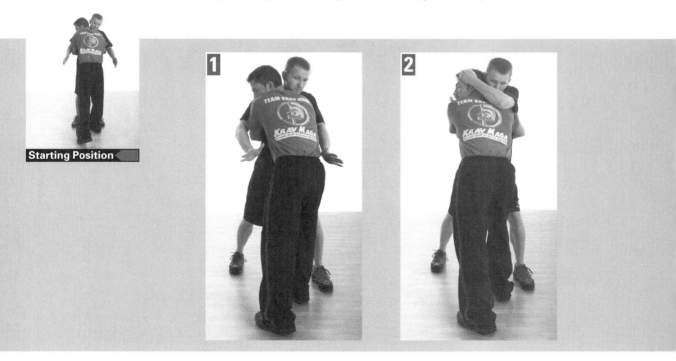

Starting Position

continued on next page

Bearhug from the Front with Arms Free (Leverage on the Neck)

continued from previous page

3 Twist the attacker's face away. His chin should rotate away from your body. You may aid this motion by placing the heel of your other palm against his chin and pushing.

4 As the attacker is peeled away, step out with your foot, allowing him to drop down. Counterattack with straight punches or hammerfist punches.

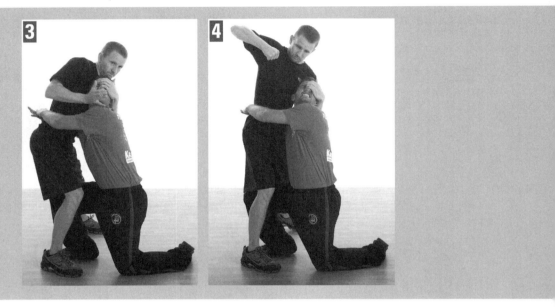

NEUTRALIZING THE ATTACKER Continue with strikes, including additional punches or hammerfists, elbows, and knees, until it's safe to disengage, then create distance.

KEY POINTS

- base and space as much as possible, although this may be difficult in this position
- reach around his head to catch at the bridge of his nose and in his eyes
- twist his chin away, "peeling" it along your body to create leverage and take him down and to the side
- attack aggressively with hammerfists, straight punches, etc.
- disengage when deemed safe

COMMONLY ASKED QUESTIONS

When should I use this technique rather than the simpler "space and base" technique?
This technique should be employed any time you cannot adequately create a base and deliver simple knee strikes.

Can I try this technique before the simpler "space and base" technique?
Yes, but as the question implies, the other technique is simpler. This technique takes slightly longer, and if the attacker intended to take you down, you are at risk.

Why should I step out with the other foot?
Stepping out allows you to take him down without having him fall on your body or leg. The body motion also adds to the power of your movement.

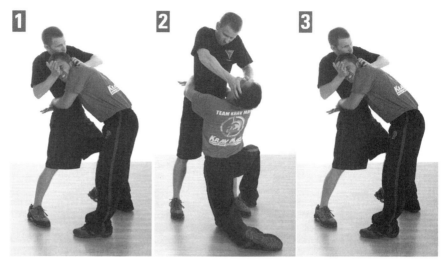

What if I cannot reach around his head to grab his face?
Excellent question. Remember that Krav Maga is principle based. The principle is to create leverage on his neck, which prevents the opponent from completing a takedown. There are a variety of ways to create that leverage, as seen in the following additional photos:

Photo 1: If the opponent's head is buried low against your body, drive the webbing of your same-side hand up under his nose, then use the other hand to help.

Photo 2: If his head is buried straight against your chest, use your fingers in his eyes.

Photo 3: If his head is turned inward toward your chest, use the same-side hand to create the leverage.

There are other examples, but it's most important to remember that you want to grab his face and tilt his chin, creating leverage on his neck to take him down.

Training Tips: The defender is very vulnerable to takedowns in this position. We're not teaching reality-based self-defense unless we acknowledge that, if the attacker closes the space this much before we react and intended to take us down, we are probably on the ground by now. That's why we train in groundfighting. However, if we're able to base out just a little, we can delay the takedown long enough to apply leverage on the neck.

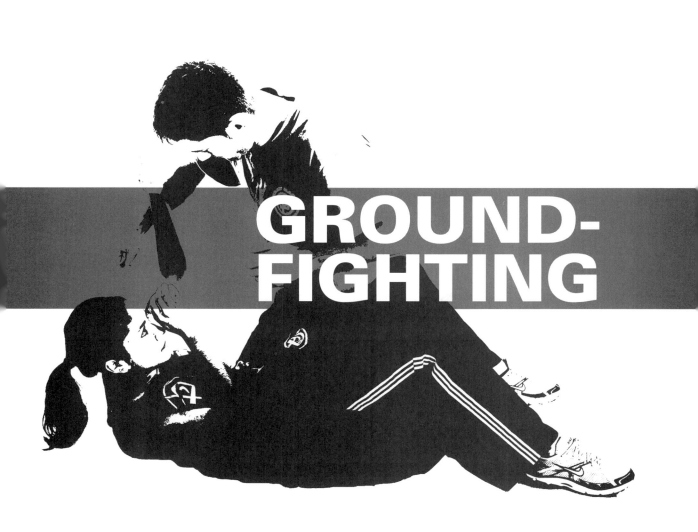

GROUND-FIGHTING

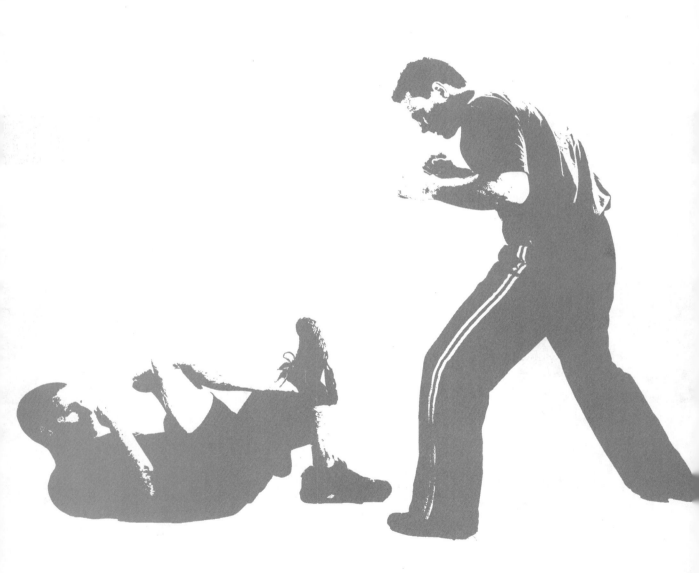

Groundfighting Overview

Groundfighting represents a significant change in any self-defense situation for a number of reasons. First, when you're on the ground, your options become limited. You cannot simply disengage and run away—you must get up first. Second, your ability to strike becomes much more limited, especially if you're on your back. Third, your opponent's weight and strength, which are factors even in a standup situation, become even more of an issue if he is on top of you. Fourth, the popularity of groundfighting, as seen in competitions such as the Ultimate Fighting Championship, increases the likelihood that your opponent may have some knowledge of these techniques. Fifth, and finally, if you're dealing with multiple assailants, some of whom may be standing, you're at an extreme disadvantage on the ground.

A Note on Biting, Gouging, and Scratching

Many advocates of reality-based self-defense and streetfighting say that "dirty" tactics such as biting, eye-gouging, and scratching are effective counter-attacks to experienced groundfighters. They are right, but only to a point. A grappler tries to maintain contact with you so he can control you. Biting him is a great way to discourage that contact. But many grapplers are clever, and he may use his superior knowledge to position himself so that he can't be bitten or scratched. Also, remember that he can bite and scratch you, too! In the end, you should consider these "dirty" tactics as valuable tools in your tool box…but they are NOT a substitute for a solid working knowledge of ground skills.

For these reasons, we do NOT want to go to the ground if we can help it, and we want to GET UP as soon as possible. However, our desire to avoid a groundfight doesn't mean we ignore this area of training. In fact, it means the opposite. We must train ourselves to be competent in groundfighting so that we can deal with the situation decisively and effectively, and then get to our feet.

In this section, you'll learn how to deal with the full mount, side mount, and guard both defensively and offensively. However, in keeping with our goal to avoid the groundfight if possible, we begin with a basic defense against a takedown.

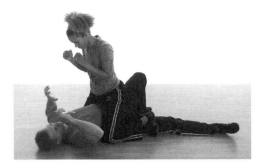

Full mount. See page 162.

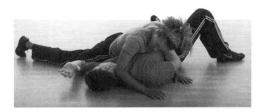

Side mount. See page 164.

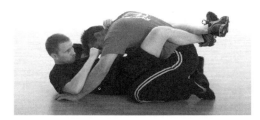

Guard. See page 167.

As we said at the outset, Krav Maga for Beginners focuses mostly on yellow and orange belt levels. We usually teach proper takedowns later in the system, simply because we don't want our students going to the ground if they don't know what to do when they get there. However, since this book covers sprawls, we do want you to learn a basic takedown so that, at the very least, you can train to sprawl against a partner who is attacking you effectively.

The takedown we teach here is very basic. In Complete Krav Maga, *it's referred to as a "Simple Takedown" and is essentially a tackle.*

Starting position: Face your partner in a left-leg-forward fighting stance.

1 Drop low and lunge forward, catching your partner around the legs with your head and/or shoulder in his stomach. Your arms may be clasped, or you can hook one hand around each leg.

2 Pull the attacker's legs in toward you and lift slightly. At the same time, use your legs to drive your weight into his stomach.

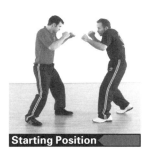

Starting Position

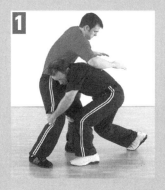

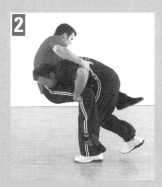

Training Tips: More effective versions of the Simple Takedown involve getting your hips in close (underneath your chest) so that the defender cannot simply push your head downward. However, this is a good, simple takedown that helps us to train our sprawling technique.

ATTACK In this attack, the attacker lunges in ("shoots," in grappling parlance) to grab the defender's legs and take him down.

IMMEDIATE DANGER *None (impact with the ground).* Similar to bearhugs, the takedown itself doesn't represent much danger, although some takedowns involve slamming the defender to the ground, so we should consider this.

SECONDARY DANGERS *Takedown, multiple attackers.* The takedown isn't a "hold" by the same definition as a bearhug. In this attack, the assailant has no intention of staying in that position. His goal is to put you on the ground immediately.

SOLUTION & INITIAL COUNTERATTACK *Sprawl, Counterattack*

1 Kick your feet back immediately, with your feet splayed wide. Drive your hips down and forward while keeping your chest up and eyes forward in the fight. This position makes it difficult for the attacker to continue driving underneath to catch your legs. As you sprawl, brace your forearms along one side of the attacker's neck and shoulders.

2 Once you feel that you've stopped his initial movement and regained your balance, deliver knee strikes.

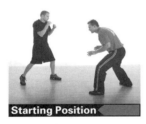

Starting Position

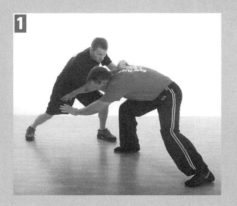

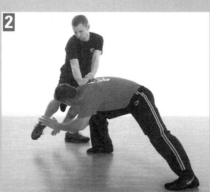

NEUTRALIZING THE ATTACKER Continue with knee strike and/or push the attacker's head to the ground, disengage, and create distance.

KEY POINTS

- sprawl by kicking your feet explosively backward
- drive your hips down, but keep your chest forward
- brace your forearms against the attacker's shoulder/neck area
- when you feel stable, deliver knees
- disengage when deemed safe

COMMONLY ASKED QUESTIONS

Why is it important to kick your feet back first?
Attackers who know how to "shoot" this way do so very quickly and with great determination. You must get your feet and legs far from them. If you have a tendency to move your hips back first and then your feet, you will get caught.

Why is it important to drive your hips downward?
Determined attackers will continue to drive forward, even when you think you're safe. Driving your hips forward and downward "blocks" them from reaching your legs. Also, if the attacker has a partial hold of your legs, this will help to break their hold.

When I brace my forearms against the attacker, should I have one arm on each side of his head, or both arms on one side?
It's better to have both arms on one side. This prevents accidental head butts and allows for easier disengagement. However, your primary goal is to stop his forward progress, so having one arm on each side of his head is better than nothing.

Training Tips: Many groundfighting experts advocate different arm positions, such as having one or both arms extended straight down to help control the attacker after the sprawl. There are both advantages and disadvantages to these variations. For our purposes, we'll simply state that we choose this position (elbows down, hands up) because it's close to the body's reflexive reaction to someone lunging at us.

A *"full mount"* is a position in which the attacker is on top, straddling the defender. Because the full mount is a dominant position, we want to maintain it as long as it's tactically desirable for us. To maintain the full mount, you must be prepared to base out whenever necessary.

1 When the attacker tries to buck you off the top position, drop your weight back into your hips, drop your chest down to your opponent's chest, and splay your hands forward and to the side.

2-3 The attacker may try to trap one of your arms when you base out so be prepared to pop up immediately. To avoid the trap, immediately and swiftly slide your elbow down toward your hip. If you simply lift your arm from the floor, you may find it trapped by his arm.

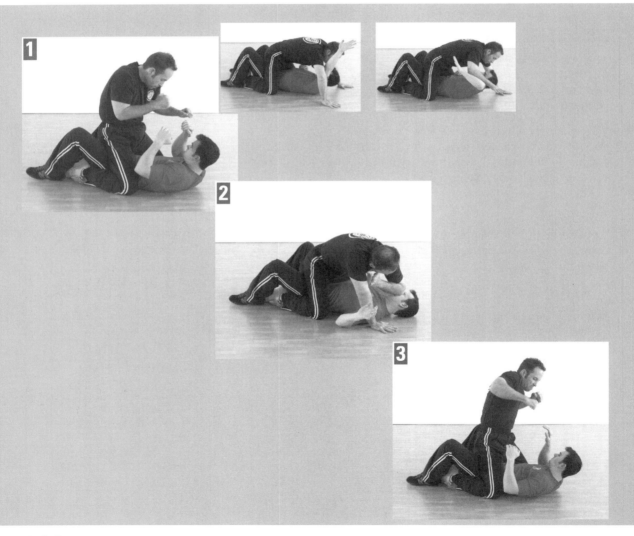

Striking from the Full Mount

When in the full mount, a number of strikes are available to you: straight punches, hook punches, hammerfists, elbows from various angles, gouging/scratching/biting, and (possibly) headbutts. Primary target areas are the face and throat. However, the issue is balance. You cannot over-commit your weight so much that you lose your balance, or so that the attacker (on the bottom) is able to reverse you.

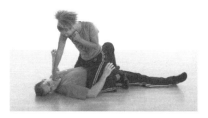

Straight punch

Straight Punches

Practice left and right straight punches (or palm heel strikes as well), put-ting just enough weight into the punch so that you can do damage, but keep your back relatively straight and some weight back in your hips.

Elbows

Drop your elbows down, but keep your weight back in your hips.

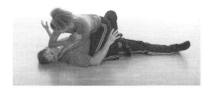

Elbow

Hammerfist Punches

Hammerfist punches, like palm heel strikes, are a viable alternative any time you worry about hitting the skull instead of the face.

Gouging/Biting/Scratching

Always a viable option here, especially when used in conjunction with other strikes. As an example, consider gouging at the eyes then, when the attacker puts his hands to his face to stop your gouging, drop an elbow down on both his hands and face.

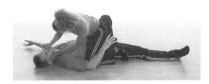

Hammerfist punch

Headbutts

Headbutts are less available from the full mount. The attacker's head will often be below the line of your head, increasing the danger that you'll strike his skull with your face. However, if your position and body type allow for it, a headbutt to his face is possible.

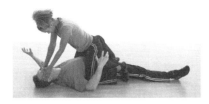

Gouging

Training Tips: It's important to practice this "strike—base out—strike" approach. Vary the rhythm so that you're not basing out predictably. Pop up immediately so that the attacker cannot trap your arm and roll you.

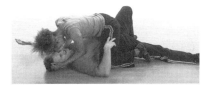

Headbutt

Side mount is, in many ways, a more advantageous position than full mount. First, it's somewhat more difficult for the person on the bottom to reverse you. Second, you can add knee strikes to your arsenal. There are two variations of the Side Mount position. One is better for control, and the other for striking.

Variation #1

1 With the attacker on the ground, sprawl your upper body over his torso. Put your weight through your chest onto his body, keeping your elbows pressed in against his body and head to keep him tight.

2 Pull your bottom knee (the one closest to his hip) up so that it presses tightly against his body, and extend the top leg (the one closest to his head) out so that your hip touches the floor.

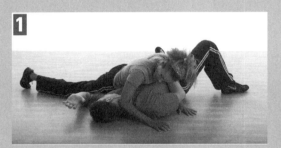
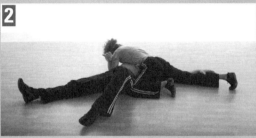

Variation #2

1 Take a position similar to Variation #1 with your upper body. However, in this variation, *both* knees come up tightly as your elbows push down and in. This position by its nature takes some of the weight off his chest, meaning he may have a little more room to escape. However, it puts you in a better position to strike. Pinch everything in tightly against the attacker so that he has as little room as possible!

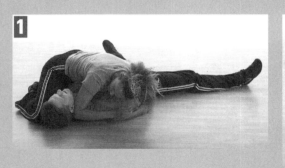
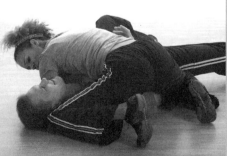

Striking from Side Mount

In conjunction with all the strikes listed below, be prepared to drop back into position quickly to keep him trapped.

Straight Punches

Practice left and right straight punches (or palm heel strikes as well) to the face, stomach, or groin.

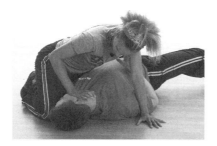

Palm heel strike

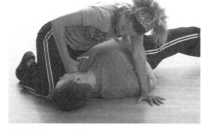

Straight punch

Elbows

Elbows to the side of his head or downward to his face are very effective.

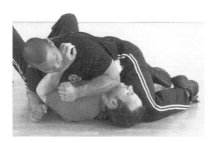

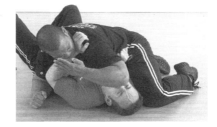

Hammerfist Punches

Hammerfists are a possibility, although from this position elbow strikes may be stronger.

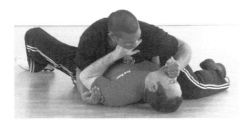

continued on next page

Striking from Side Mount

continued from previous page

Biting/Gouging/Scratching

Gouging and scratching at the face may be extremely effective here, especially because one or both of his arms may be trapped away from his face by your body position. If he puts one arm up to push your upper body away, you can bite.

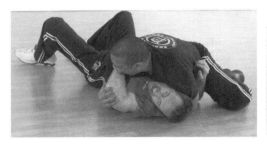 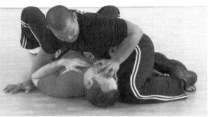

Headbutts

Headbutts are somewhat more available from this position than a full mount because your head will be "lower" relative to his face.

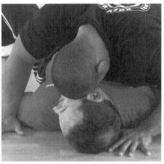

Knees

Deliver knees to his head or body by raising your leg away from him and then driving the knee in explosively.

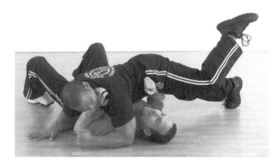

Training Tips: As stated, practice delivering a strike and then immediately reestablishing your position. Any time you raise a limb to strike, you create space that he may use to try an escape.

Operating When You Have Someone in the Guard

When you're on your back with your legs wrapped around the opponent, this is called the "guard" position. While you're still in a somewhat defensive position, you're much better off than if the attacker were in the full mount. You can exert some control over him with your legs and, later, learn submission techniques such as arm bars and triangle chokes.

There are two basic choices when it comes to applying a guard position. **Closed guard** means your ankles are crossed and knees are apart. This hold is designed to control your opponent. **Open guard** involves keeping your feet apart and knees closer together. This hold is designed to offer you more options to kick your opponent away or control him.

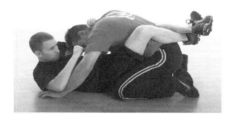

Closed guard

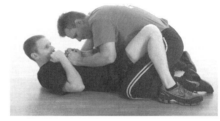

Open guard

Using Your Legs

At this level, one of our primary goals is to learn to control the opponent as much as possible. When the attacker tries to sit back so he can punch, use your legs to pull him in close. When the attacker tries to get close to stifle your punches, use your legs and hips to push him away. Overall, use this "push/pull" combination to disrupt his balance.

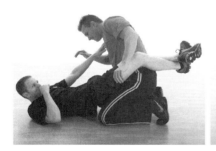

Control by pushing the attacker away with your hips and legs.

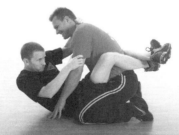

Control by pulling the attacker in with your legs.

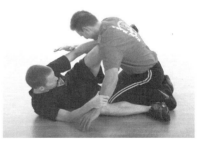

Use your legs and hips to transition into another position, escape, or attack.

Striking from your back can be difficult because it's harder to generate power. However, a few strikes are possible, as follows:

Straight Punches

If the attacker exposes his face, send a straight punch. Be sure to rotate your shoulder and use your hip to create as much power as possible. Since your legs are wrapped around his waist, use the attacker as a base to help generate power.

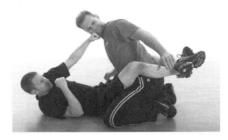

Straight punch

Elbows

Sometimes the attacker will bring his head in close. Elbow #1 to his jaw or Elbow #7 to the back of his head or clavicle can be very effective.

Biting/Gouging/Scratching

These techniques can be very effective when the attacker is close. Tear at the face and gouge the eyes. Catch the hair (if any) and face, and twist the neck.

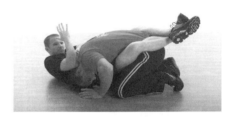

Elbow strike

Training Tips: There is value in learning to strike from any position. However, as stated, it's much more difficult to strike from your back. Later in the system, you'll learn submission/grappling techniques that are more effective from this position.

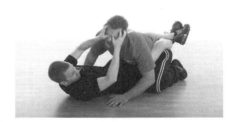

Gouging

Kicking Off from the Guard

This is a basic escape when you find yourself on your back with someone in your guard.

Starting position: You have your opponent in your guard.

1 Shift to one hip, bringing your top knee in so that your shin presses against his body. Your hands should be up to protect against punches.

2-3 Kick your bottom foot against his hip to create space, then kick your top foot against his chest or face. Be sure to extend your hip during both kicks. Get up and create distance.

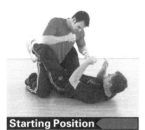

Starting Position

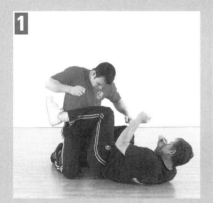

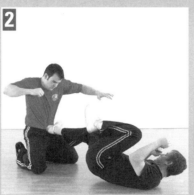

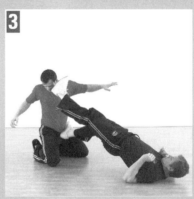

Training Tips: It's important to shift to one hip in order to perform the technique, especially if you lack flexibility. Turning to one hip makes it easier to bring the top knee in against the attacker's body, which helps to create distance for the second kick.

Just as we can use our legs to manipulate someone else while they're in our guard, the attacker may try to manipulate us if we're in his guard. As you become a more proficient groundfighter, you'll learn a number of techniques to strike from and escape from the guard. At this level, we present basic and effective techniques that will keep you safe and allow you to neutralize the attacker.

Variation #1: Basic position (close position)

If you find yourself in the attacker's guard, your first job is to establish a basic position to avoid being attacked or reversed.

1 Kneel with your knees fairly wide and your toes curled so that you're on the balls of your feet (not the shoe laces). Press your chest and head against his chest and put your hands on his biceps to limit his strikes and other attacks.

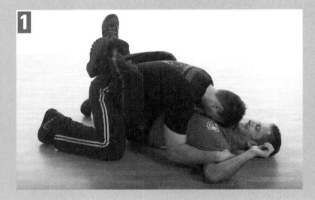

Variation #2: Sitting-up position

1 If you want to get to a position that allows you to strike more effectively, sit back inside his guard, keeping your weight in your heels. Tuck your elbows in tight, with your hands grabbing at the area of his belt buckle.

2 From here, deliver strikes to the face or groin.

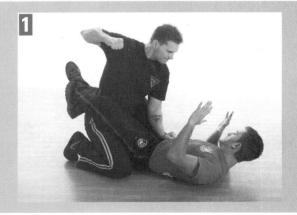
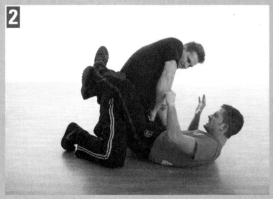

Training Tip: Be all the way in or all the way out. Even if you're not familiar with basic "submission" attacks such as arm bars or triangles, you can learn some basic principles that protect you from these attacks. One of these principles is this: Be all the way in or all the way out.

If you want to get close to the attacker, get *very* close, with your head up near his chest and shoulders, your arms and shoulders in very deep, and your hips pressed against the backs of his thighs. This makes it more difficult for him to move his hips and legs up high enough to attack you.

If you want to create distance from the attacker, get *very* far out so that your elbows are below the line of his groin and your head and shoulders are high up away from him. This makes it hard for him to reach you, and makes it easier for you to slide out if he tries a submission-type attack.

As with the other areas we've discussed, the strikes here are not new. Straight punches, elbows, headbutts, bite/gouge/scratch, and hammerfists are all possible.

As with striking while in the full mount, you must be very cognizant of your balance. A smart attacker will use his legs to push you away or pull you in when you try to strike in an attempt to take your balance away. Always operate from a solid base, and do not compromise this base for anything.

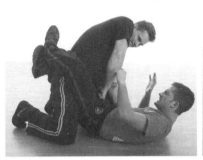

Straight punch

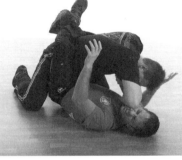

Elbow strike

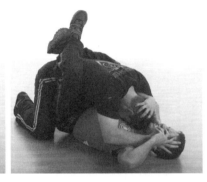

Gouging

Training Tip: Never overextend your arms. One of the basic attacks from the guard is an arm bar, in which the opponent traps one arm and can break it. You expose yourself to an arm bar if you extend one arm too far and let him trap it. Practice punching and recoiling quickly, always bringing your elbows in tight and close to you; this makes an arm bar very difficult to perform.

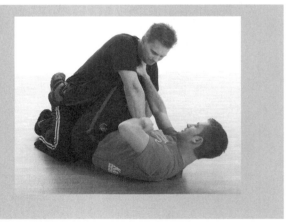

There are a number of guard escapes, including stacking and passing the guard, but again, this book focuses on the basics. The simplest way to escape the guard is to sit back and strike the groin.

Starting position: The attacker holds you close so that you cannot strike effectively.

1 Use eye gouges, scratching, and biting to create distance.

2 Sit up, keep your back straight, and strike down to the groin.

3 When the attacker pulls his knees in to protect his groin, sit back further, putting your hands on his legs to prevent him from kicking you.

4 Stand up and back up to create distance.

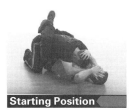

Starting Position

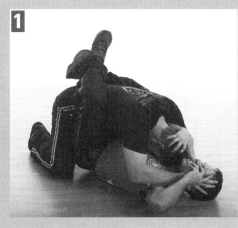

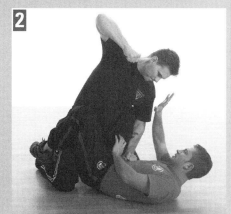

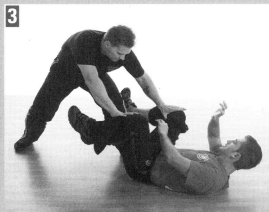

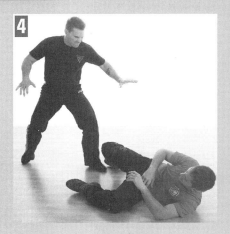

continued on next page

Escape from the Guard

continued from previous page

Training Tips: Whether the attacker holds you in close or not, he has two basic choices for a guard position. You have two guard positions to choose from: closed guard and open guard.

If the attacker chooses an open guard, you should be able to sit back, create distance, and get away.

If the attacker chooses a closed guard, his crossed ankles will prevent you from simply sliding away from him. However, if his ankles are crossed, his groin will be exposed. Strike hard to the groin, which will usually cause him to open his guard and bring his knees in to protect his groin. At this point, you can get up and away.

Dealing with the Full Mount

Earlier, we discussed how to maintain our position when we're in the full mount. Now, we must defend our-selves when the attacker is on top of us. There are two basic ways to deal with this situation.

Starting position: The attacker has you in full mount.

1 Dig your elbows into his thighs and keep your hands up to protect your face. Pull your feet up close to your butt. Your goal is to keep the attacker low on your hips, where your movements will affect him. Do *not* let the attacker scoot up onto your chest with his knees under your armpits. This makes everything much more difficult for you: your arms become trapped, and your hip action does not affect him at all.

If the attacker does manage to scoot up, try jamming your elbows into his thighs and wriggling upward so that he ends up back down near your hips.

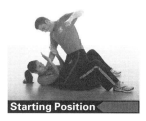

Starting Position

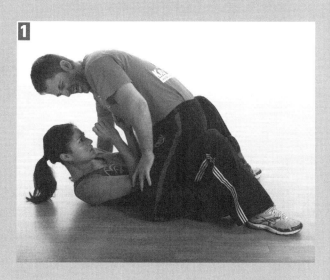

Training Tips: In general from the position, do not extend your arms upward. This exposes them to several types of sub-mission-style attacks, such as an arm bar. Keep your elbows bent and close to you.

The basic principles for defending against strikes are the same here as when standing.

Keep your chin tucked and your head off the ground. You should use Inside Defenses and 360° Defenses to block straight punches and outside attacks such as hook punches. If the attacker uses an elbow, you may need to defend it with two arms rather than one.

In addition, buck your hips. Every time the attacker tries to throw a punch, buck your hips to disturb his balance. At the very least, you'll weaken his punch. At most, you may cause him to base out so that he cannot punch until he recovers.

Training Tips: Try a basic drill where your partner sits in full mount and tries to punch. Every time he punches, buck your hips. Try to time the hip action so that it coincides with the beginning of the punch for maximum affect. This is harder to do during a real fight, but it's a great drill to develop awareness in this position.

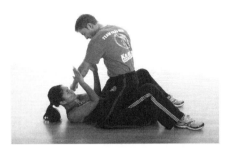

Inside defense

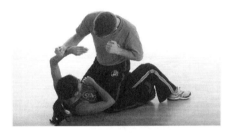

360° defense

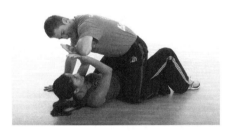

Defend an elbow strike with two arms.

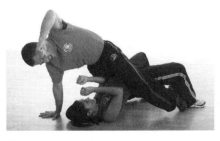

Buck your hips to upset attacker's balance.

Trap and Roll

Starting position: The attacker has you in full mount.

1 Buck your hips to make the attacker base out.

2-3 With one arm, reach out to trap one of his arms. You can reach either over (trapping from the inside out) or under (trapping from the outside in). Generally, reaching over the arm makes for a better hold but may take longer to execute. Be sure that you trap the arm above the elbow so that he cannot slide his elbow out.

4 Using your leg, trap the attacker's leg on the same side as the arm—as much as possible at the same time as you trap the arm. Buck your hips again, driving upward toward your head.

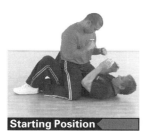

Starting Position

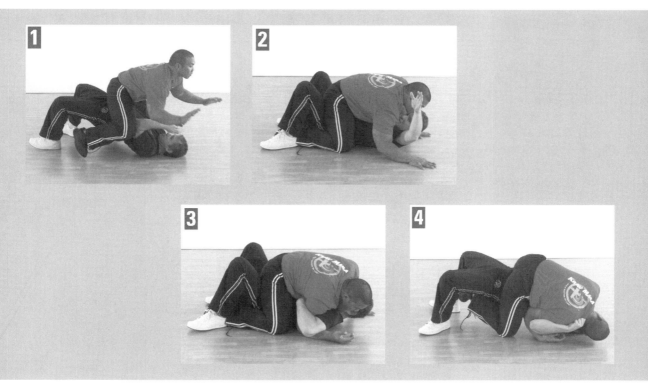

continued on next page

GROUNDFIGHTING **177**

continued from previous page

5-7 At the end of this motion, roll your hips over toward the trapped side. Drive over with your feet to end up on top, striking as you go. Your goal should be to deliver an elbow to the face, but if the attacker's resistance makes that impossible, deliver groin strikes.

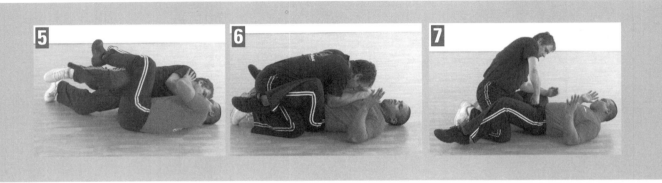

Training Tips: When you buck your hips (also called bridging), do it explosively. You do not want to give the attacker time to react or adjust. Also, do NOT roll sideways. Buck your hips toward your head, then roll the attacker over your shoulder. Rolling sideways will not give you the same power or degree of movement.

When trapping the arm, there are a variety of alternatives. We have described two here, but in the end, trap the arm any way you can. If the attacker is wearing thick clothing, you can reach up and grab his clothes, pulling his arm in close. If he is holding his hand in the air, reach up and grab that hand with your two hands. The method of trapping is not important, so long as you trap his arm effectively!

Trapping his arm prevents him from "posting" that hand out when you try to roll him over. If he is able to post his arm out, he will stop you from rolling and you will end up back where you started.

Finally, be aware that you are in a difficult position. It may take several attempts to successfully trap his arm. Do not panic, but do not give up, either. Every time he tries to strike you, buck your hips. At the very least, you will affect his balance and make it harder for him to strike. At most, you will create another opportunity for the trap and roll.

Elbow Escape (Shrimping)

This technique does not reverse the attacker, but takes you from being fully mounted to a guard position, which is more advantageous for you. For the sake of clarity, we'll assume we're turning to the left first. You can, of course, go to the opposite side first if you prefer.

Starting position: The attacker has you in full mount.

1 With the attacker in a full mount, shift onto your left hip and wedge your left elbow between your body and the attacker's right knee to create space. You can use your right hand to help push the attacker up and away.

2 With your left leg extended and flat on the floor and the right foot flat on the floor, push ("shrimp" in grappling parlance) your hips to the right side. Use your abs to help pull your hips up and out. Your right hand can assist by helping push the attacker's right knee away.

3 There should now be space between the attacker's right knee and your body. Bending your left knee, slide that leg up and out (it may slide under the attacker's right leg, which is fine). Keep that left leg flat on the floor as it slides up, or it may bump into the attacker's leg or body.

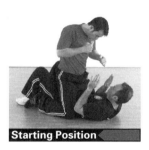

Starting Position

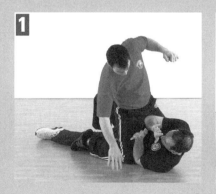

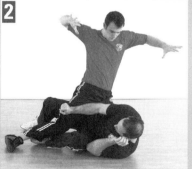

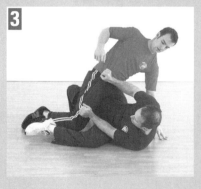

continued on next page

Elbow Escape (Shrimping)

continued from previous page

4 Once that leg is out, wrap it around the attacker's leg, then switch to the other hip.

5-6 Perform the same movement on that side, and wrap both legs around the attacker. You now have him in your guard. If you have created a great deal of space during this movement, you can simply kick off rather than put him in your guard.

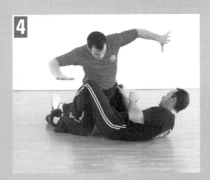
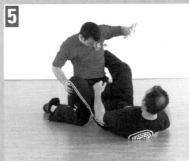
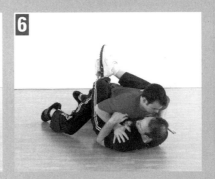

Training Tips: This description says to wedge your left elbow between his knee and your body. You can use your left hand, if you prefer.

Two simultaneous actions create the space: pushing away on the attacker's knee and pulling your hips up and out. Make sure you do both.

Focus on pushing the attacker's knee *away*, not upward. He may be too heavy to lift. However, if the knee lifts up a little, this can help you to slide your leg out.

Defense against Choke while Full Mounted

The attacker, in a full mount, may try to choke you instead of punching. The defense here is a combination of two techniques you already know: first, the plucking defense against a choke while standing; second, the trap and roll principle you've already learned.

Starting position: The attacker tries to choke you from a full mount.

1-2 With the attacker straddling you and with his hands on your throat, pluck his hands from your throat and trap them to your shoulders. At the same time, bring one foot up to trap one of his legs.

3-4 Buck your hips up to throw the attacker up and forward, then tilt him over one shoulder (the same side as the leg you have trapped). Note that your hands, having trapped his hands to your shoulders, should keep him from basing out.

5 Roll the attacker over and immediately counterattack with an elbow to the face, or other available strikes. Disengage and get up as soon as possible.

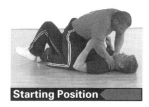

Starting Position

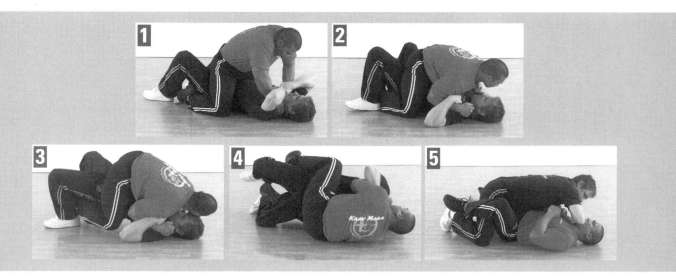

Training Tips: Note that the range of motion of your pluck may be limited by the floor. You should still be able to relieve enough pressure from your throat to allow you to trap and roll.

Defense against Close Choke or Headlock while Full Mounted

The attacker, in a full mount, may try to choke you while bending his arms and leaning in close, or put you in a headlock. Because his body is so close to you, you may not be able to pluck.

Starting position: The attacker puts you in a headlock while in a full mount.

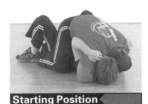 As the attacker comes in close, wrap your arm around one of his arms to trap it into place. If the attack is a headlock, trap the arm that is wrapped around your neck. Trap the leg on the same side as the arm you have trapped, and execute a trap and roll. You'll most likely end up in the attacker's guard. If the attack was a headlock, the attacker's arm may still be wrapped around your neck.

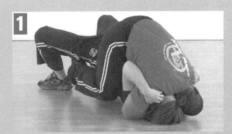

Starting Position

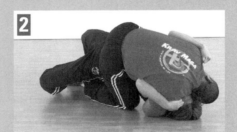

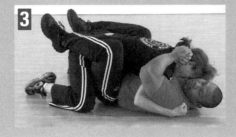

4-6 Push the blade of your arm across his face (a "crossface") to force him to let go, then continue with counterattacks.

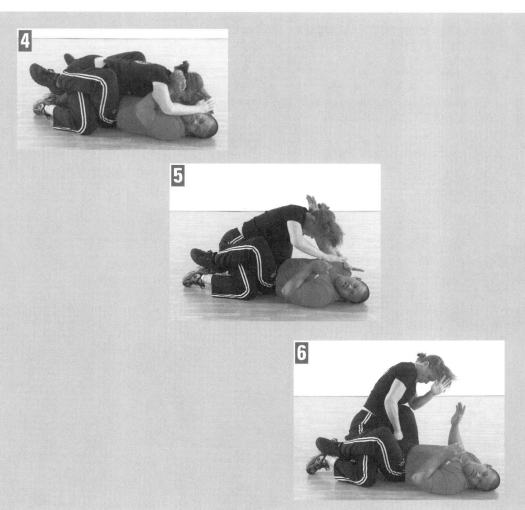

Training Tips: Ultimately, you should try to roll the attacker to the side where you feel most of his weight. However, feeling this does take some time and experience. In general, just remember to trap the arm that is wrapped around your neck if you are in a headlock, and trap the arm on the same side as the attacker's head if you're in a close choke.

Getting Up from the Ground

At the end of all groundfighting techniques mentioned here, it's important to get up as soon as possible. The following is a safe technique for getting up from your back. Note that this technique provides you with both a defensive and offensive tool as you stand up.

1 Assume your attacker has backed off, perhaps in response to a kick. Bring yourself up to a modified sitting position, keeping your base foot on the ground, your kicking foot up, and one hand on the same side as the base foot up defensively. Your other hand should be on the ground for support. Your kicking foot should be ready to stomp outward.

2-4 Using your base foot and your base hand, lift your hips off the ground. Quickly swing your kicking foot beneath you (think of swinging your hip back at an angle). As you do, place your foot well behind you, not directly beneath you.

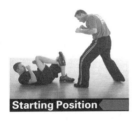

Starting Position

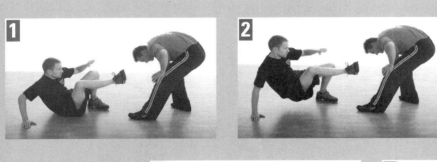

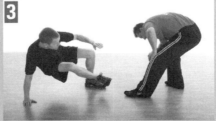

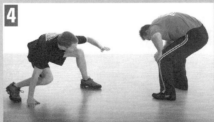

5 Stand up, taking a few steps backward to increase the distance.

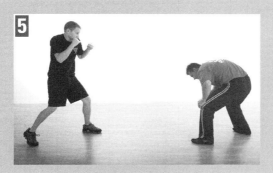

Training Tips: As stated, swing your foot and your hip on a diagonal rather than straight back. This requires less flexibility. If you cannot lift your hips off the ground with just one hand, you can use two. Just be aware that you're less protected this way.

Be aware that if your opponent is standing too close, he may be able to punch or kick you as you try to rise. In general, make sure there is at least a little distance between you before you try to get up.

Index

Other Ulysses Press Books

Complete Krav Maga: The Ultimate Guide to Over 230 Self-Defense and Combative Techniques
Darren Levine & John Whitman, $21.95
Developed for the Israel military forces, Krav Maga has gained an international reputation as an easy-to-learn yet highly effective art of self-defense. Clearly written and extensively illustrated, *Complete Krav Maga* details every aspect of the system including hand-to-hand combat moves and weapons defense techniques.

Forza: The Samurai Sword Workout
Ilaria Montagnani, $14.95
Transforms sword-fighting techniques into a program that combines the excitement of sword play with a heart-pumping, full-body workout.

Functional Training for Athletes at All Levels: Workouts for Agility, Speed, and Power
James C. Radcliffe, $15.95
Teaches all athletes the functional training exercises that will produce the best results in their sport by mimicking the actual movements they utilize in that sport. With these unique programs, athletes can simultaneously improve posture, balance, stability, and mobility.

Get Firefighter Fit: The Complete Workout from the Former Director of the New York City Fire Department Physical Training Program
Kevin S. Malley with David K. Spierer, $15.95
Using a four-phase progressive approach to total body conditioning, *Get Firefighter Fit* presents a comprehensive training method that has proven successful in transforming out-of-shape rookies into top-flight firefighters.

The Martial Artist's Book of Yoga: Improve Flexibility, Balance and Strength for Higher Kicks, Faster Strikes, Smoother Throws, Safer Falls, and Stronger Stances

Lily Chou with Kathe Rothacher, $14.95

A great training supplement for martial artists, this book clearly illustrates how specific yoga poses can directly improve one's martial arts abilities.

Plyometrics for Athletes at All Levels: A Training Guide for Explosive Speed and Power

Neal Pire, $15.95

Provides the nonprofessional with an easy-to-understand explanation of why plyometrics works, the sports-training research behind it, and how to integrate plyometrics into an overall fitness program.

The Secret Art of Pressure Point Fighting: Techniques to Disable Anyone in Seconds Using Minimal Force

Vince Morris, $15.95

Martial arts legends tell of masters who can defeat an opponent with one blow. *The Secret Art of Pressure Point Fighting* transforms the myth into a modern, anatomically based self-defense technique that allows smaller defenders to defeat larger attackers by striking at the vulnerable points on their bodies.

Special Ops Fitness Training: High-Intensity Workouts of Navy SEALs, Delta Force, Marine Force Recon, and Army Rangers

Mark De Lisle, $14.95

Drawn from the actual programs used by America's special operation forces (Navy SEALs, Delta Force, Marine Force Recon, and Army Rangers), recognized fitness expert, author, and ex-Navy SEAL Mark De Lisle challenges readers with some of the most rigorous training employed by anyone, anywhere.

Total Heart Rate Training: Customize and Maximize Your Workout Using a Heart Rate Monitor

Joe Friel, $15.95

Shows anyone participating in aerobic sports, from novice to expert, how to increase the effectiveness of his or her workout by utilizing a heart rate monitor.

Workouts from Boxing's Greatest Champs

Gary Todd, $14.95

Features dramatic photos, workout secrets, and behind-the-scenes details of Muhammad Ali, Roy Jones, Jr., Fernando Vargas, and other legends.

To order these books call 800-377-2542 or 510-601-8301, fax 510-601-8307, e-mail ulysses@ulyssespress.com, or write to Ulysses Press, P.O. Box 3440, Berkeley, CA 94703. All retail orders are shipped free of charge. California residents must include sales tax. Allow two to three weeks for delivery.

About the Authors
and Photographer

Darren Levine, a 6th-degree black belt, is the founder of the nonprofit Krav Maga Association and serves as the Chief Executive Officer and U.S. Chief Instructor of Krav Maga Worldwide. He has trained thousands of civilians and hundreds of law enforcement and military personnel around the world. In addition, Darren is a Deputy District Attorney who has won the California Deputy District Attorney of the Year Award. Darren has lectured widely on use-of-force issues and is well-known in the law enforcement community. In the Los Angeles District Attorney's office, he serves as a senior member of the Crimes Against Peace Officers Section (CAPOS), an elite unit that prosecutes offenders who murder, or attempt to murder, police officers. In his dual roles as Krav Maga Chief Instructor and as a Deputy District Attorney, he has dedicated his life to the safety of others.

John Whitman is a 4th-degree black belt in Krav Maga and the former president of Krav Maga Worldwide. He holds instructor's diplomas from both the Krav Maga Association of America and Wingate University in Israel, and has trained at the Israeli Military Institute in personal protection and installation protection. John has been teaching Krav Maga since 1994, and has trained thousands of civilians as well as law enforcement and military units, including the Air Force Office of Special Investigations Antiterrorist Specialty Team and the Special Operations Group for the Japanese Self-Defense Force. John has also published a number of books, including several *24* novels. He is the co-founder and CEO of Focus Self Defense and Fitness.

Ryan Hoover is the owner of one of six Krav Maga Worldwide Regional Training Centers. He owns multiple centers in North Carolina, operating as Ryan Hoover's Extreme Karate and Fit to Fight. The recipient of the first ever "Fighting Spirit" award presented by Krav Maga Worldwide, he has been training in Krav Maga since 2001 and is one of a small group of trainers within the organization authorized to train and certify others as Krav Maga Worldwide instructors. Ryan is also a member of the KMW licensee advisory board and a KMW Advanced Force Training Instructor.

Andy Mogg is a well-known and much-published photographer. Born in England in 1954, he worked as a consultant, then writer and photographer. At 17, he moved from London to Belgium, traveling and working his way through Europe; he settled in ~~3 1901 04581 2833~~ ow runs a thriving photography studio in Oakland, California. For more ~~...~~ w.dancingimages.com.